**This book belongs to the OutCenter
resource library of Berrien County**

Please return to:
OutCenter
132 Water Street
Benton Harbor, MI 49022
E-mail : info@outcenter.org
269-925-8330

Kathleen A. Dolan, PhD

Lesbian Women and Sexual Health
The Social Construction of Risk and Susceptibility

*Pre-publication
REVIEWS,
COMMENTARIES,
EVALUATIONS . . .*

"Dolan's groundbreaking study of 162 self-identified lesbians is an innovative and methodologically solid piece of scholarship. Through her triangulation of several methods—including in-depth interviews, focus groups and quantitative surveys—this grounded theory monograph brilliantly captures the range of variation in lesbian identities, health-seeking beliefs, and wellness practices. The presentation of previously underrepresented data is a boon for the field, as is the author's incisive interpretive analysis.

This work is especially significant for its engagement with complexities. First, Dolan accurately illustrates the emergent process of identifying as lesbian and does not merely accept previous social scientific categories of sexual identity as stable or taken for granted. Her research demonstrates how her informants, even though they express fluidity in their actions and self-identifications, simultaneously reinforce static definitions of sexual identity. Second, her interpretation of the data spans both the microsociological aspects of human symbolic interaction as well as the macrosociological policy implications of health care organization and delivery. Third, this dynamic monograph fills a research gap and can be used as a model for comprehensive studies of previously underrepresented groups."

Lisa Jean Moore, PhD, MPH
*Associate Professor of Sociology,
The College of Staten Island/
The Graduate Center/
City University of New York*

More pre-publication
REVIEWS, COMMENTARIES, EVALUATIONS . . .

"This book about lesbian perceptions of risk does a very convincing and thorough job of showing the complexities with which lesbians view sexual and other HIV and STI risks. It shows that these views are socially embedded and also that they change over time, both for the individual and for lesbian communities. For me, it is particularly striking that her sample—ten percent of whom report that they have injected illicit drugs—seems unaware of the phenomenally high risk of becoming infected with HIV facing those lesbians who inject drugs (even when compared to other injection-drug users)."

Samuel R. Friedman, PhD
Senior Research Associate,
Institute for AIDS Research;
Director of Social Theory Core,
Center for Drug Use and HIV Research,
National Development and Research
Institutes, Inc.; Senior Associate,
Department of Epidemiology,
Bloomsberg School of Public Health,
The Johns Hopkins University

The Haworth Press®
New York • London • Oxford

Lesbian Women and Sexual Health
The Social Construction of Risk and Susceptibility

Haworth Psychosocial Issues of HIV/AIDS
R. Dennis Shelby, PhD
Editor

Lesbian Women and Sexual Health
The Social Construction of Risk and Susceptibility

Kathleen A. Dolan, PhD

The Haworth Press®
New York • London • Oxford

For more information on this book or to order, visit
http://www.haworthpress.com/store/product.asp?sku=5183

or call 1-800-HAWORTH (800-429-6784) in the United States and Canada
or (607) 722-5857 outside the United States and Canada

or contact orders@HaworthPress.com

The Haworth Press, Inc., 10 Alice Street, Binghamton, NY 13904-1580.

PUBLISHER'S NOTE
Identities and circumstances of individuals discussed in this book have been changed to protect confidentiality.

Cover design by Lora Wiggins.

Library of Congress Cataloging-in-Publication Data

Dolan, Kathleen A., 1968-
    Lesbian women and sexual health : the social construction of risk and susceptibility / Kathleen A. Dolan.
        p. cm.
    Includes bibliographical references and index.
    ISBN-13: 978-0-7890-2478-7 (hc. : alk. paper)
    ISBN-10: 0-7890-2478-0 (hc. : alk. paper)
    ISBN-13: 978-0-7890-2479-4 (pbk. : alk. paper)
    ISBN-10: 0-7890-2479-9 (pbk. : alk. paper)
    1. Lesbians—Health and hygiene. 2. Lesbians—Sexual behavior. 3. Hygiene, Sexual. 4. Sexually transmitted diseases—Risk factors. 5. AIDS (Disease)—Risk factors. 6. Safe sex in AIDS prevention.
    [DNLM: 1. Homosexuality, Female. 2. Women's Health. 3. Data Collection. 4. Risk. 5. Sexually Transmitted Diseases—transmission. WA 309 D659L 2005] I. Title.

RA564.87.D654 2005
613.9'5'086643—dc22

                                                                                2004021699

Dedicated to the women
who shared their stories.

ABOUT THE AUTHOR

Kathleen A. Dolan, PhD, is Assistant Professor of Sociology at North Georgia College and State University in Dahlonega, Georgia. She received her doctorate from Georgia State University. In 1998, Dr. Dolan received a grant from the Atlanta/Emory Center for AIDS Research to study HIV/AIDS among lesbian women, which led to the creation of this book. Her previous work has been published in journals that include *Social Science & Medicine* and *Drug Use & Misuse*. Her research and teaching interests include medical sociology, substance abuse, sexuality, and mental health.

CONTENTS

Foreword

When, as a novice AIDS activist in 1987—we were all novices then—I tried to prepare an information leaflet for lesbians about safer sex and the risks of woman-to-woman transmission of HIV, I was forced to concede defeat. There was, quite simply, no information available that I could draw upon. This was the year in which Cindy Patton and Janis Kelly published their comprehensive and approachable handbook *Making It: A Woman's Guide to Sex in the Age of AIDS,* but I had no way of knowing this. It is easy to forget just how precious and rare a commodity safe-sex information was in those beleagured times, when the Internet was still the province of geeks and boffins and when U.S. President Ronald Reagan had yet to say the word "AIDS" in public.

In 1984, Her Majesty's Customs in Britain raided the only gay bookshop in the land, London's Gay's the Word, seizing safer-sex materials imported from the States and bringing 100 criminal charges against the directors. One minister was reduced to smuggling safe-sex information into the country in his diplomatic bag in order to avoid it being impounded by customs officers. The National Blood Transfusion Service refused to accept donated blood from lesbians, on the premise that homosexuality itself was somehow risky, and the British government, under Margaret Thatcher, was busy dreaming up Section 28 of the 1988 Local Government Act, prohibiting schools from "promoting homosexuality" by teaching young people anything at all about same-sex relationships. Lesbians were being told that we were both at risk and a danger to others, while being prevented from getting access to the information which might help us protect ourselves. Dark days indeed.

As I write this at the start of 2005, things have changed beyond recognition. Despite the reelection of the fiercely gay-hostile administration of George W. Bush, partnership rights and other lesbian and gay civil rights issues are firmly on the U.S. political agenda, while human rights legislation from the European Union has forced the

British government to outlaw discrimination on grounds of sexual orientation. There now exists a massive body of information about lesbian health issues, and the medical profession—always deeply conservative—has been obliged to acknowledge that some of their patients might actually be lesbians, and that their sexuality does not justify substandard or negligent care.

For me, three recent events have indicated just how profound a change this has been. The first was the publication in 1999 of Solarz' *Lesbian Health: Current Assessment and Directions for the Future* for the National Institute of Medicine. The second was that I was invited in 2003 to contribute a chapter on lesbian health to a revised version of the standard textbook on gynecology. The third was receiving the manuscript of this book, *Lesbian Women and Sexual Health: The Social Construction of Risk and Susceptibility.* At last, clinicians, nurses, and other health care workers can no longer claim ignorance as a reason to provide poor quality care or advice to their lesbian patients. The material is now in the textbooks (though this is no guarantee that it will be sensitively taught in medical schools or in nurse training), and a substantial body of information about lesbian health is now available to all.

Often the most difficult and challenging aspect for health care providers to deal with is the sheer complexity of the relationships between sexual practice, sexual identity, and sexual health. Professionals accustomed to dealing in terms of *quantifiability*—the incidence of certain diseases in certain identifiable population groups or the statistical correlation between behavior and infection—are ill equipped to deal with lesbians. As Kathleen Dolan makes clear in her research, "lesbian" means whatever any particular lesbian wants it to mean. It may mean something different, even to that individual woman, in different circumstances, and it does not have a clear-cut link to behavior—even sexual behavior. It is simply not possible to make this degree of relativity fit into the cognitive frameworks of Western scientific medicine.

That is the important contribution made by this book. Dolan and I would disagree about many things (I think, for example, that lesbians who conclude that latex gloves and dental dams are not for them are often being quite rational about risk), but her book succeeds in giving the reader a textured and nuanced picture of the complexity of lesbian sexuality and identity. This is a difficult achievement. Partly it is achieved by her methodological expertise and ingenuity—to see elements of social constructionism, symbolic interactionism, and grounded theory being used in such a pragmatic and effective way is a real delight—and partly it is achieved by the clarity with which she allows her participants to speak.

This is not a "representative" group of lesbians. No fewer than 88 percent of them have been tested for HIV, which suggests an unusual degree of awareness or of risk perception. As Dolan herself makes clear, however, there can be no "representative sample" of the "lesbian population," because those terms quickly become meaningless in the context of this complex, fluid, contingent set of experiences. The strength of her book is that it enables a reader unused to dealing with this degree of complexity not only to comprehend it, but to understand that it is possible (and necessary) to design and deliver health education and health care programs that take into account the real circumstances of women's lives. I hope that it will be widely read.

Tamsin Wilton, DPhil, MSc, PGCE
Professor of Human Sexuality
University of the West of England

Preface

The idea for this study came from my personal life. I had just recently begun dating again after a long-term relationship, and I wondered what, if any, risk I was at for sexually transmitted infections (STIs). When I started to look for information about lesbians and STIs (this was around 1998) I found that there really was not a lot out there, nor did my doctor have much information. I saw that academic articles were beginning to pop up in the literature (see Chapter 1) and decided to work from there to find out for myself just what was going on with lesbian women and sexual health.

I lived in a very diverse city with a large lesbian population and, through other research on which I had been working, I had access to women from very different backgrounds. The women in this book represent many facets of society. Their experiences and choices are influenced not only by their sexuality but also by larger issues such as race and social class, which moderate every other facet of our lives. We make choices within the contexts in which we live. These are real women, living real lives, making the best choices they know how with what they have. Although as a researcher I might conclude that some choices are less than rational or potentially unhealthy, as a person I understand that sometimes those are still the best choices. Love, trust, relationship, community, and willingness to risk impact the decisions individuals make. The women in this study candidly provide insight into their lived experiences, which in turn may provide insight for others.

Acknowledgments

The Atlanta/Emory Center for AIDS Research (CFAR) provided funding for this study.

I am grateful to Phil Davis for guidance, mentoring, and friendship. Dawn Baunach and Wendy Simonds provided essential support and feedback. Claire Sterk, friend, mentor, and teacher, is invaluable to my progress as a researcher and a person.

I am grateful for the women who worked on this study: Kim Lupo, Lisa Diedrich, Jennifer Badeaux, Brooke Silverthorne, Carranne Fields, and Stephani Shope.

I want to thank my best friend, Ketta, Melanie, my father, Laurie, Grandma, and Peter for their encouragement and support.

To Natalie, who provided me with the inspiration and fuel to write the last 100 pages of my dissertation, thank you.

Chapter 1

Introduction

It is unclear how and to what extent lesbian women are at risk for sexually transmitted infections (STIs) or human immunodeficiency virus (HIV). It is also unclear whether they perceive themselves to be at risk or how much they even think about it. For Elanor, a respondent in this study, STIs were not something she ever really thought about until she discovered she had contracted genital herpes from a female partner.

Elanor is a twenty-seven-year-old artist and waitress who identified as a lesbian: She preferred to have sex with women only and had not had sex with a man in over a year at the time of our interview. She said she did not have sex with a man during the time she believes she became infected with herpes. Elanor expressed disappointment at contracting an STI from another woman, who she said denied having herpes at the time of the sexual relationship and also when confronted. In fact, no woman or man that Elanor had ever had sex with had ever admitted to having an STI. Elanor had a college degree, worked full-time, and described herself as middle class. She was single, with no children, and had never been pregnant.

After contracting genital herpes, Elanor started asking potential sexual partners about HIV and STIs, and said she always disclosed her herpes infection before having sex with someone. In good health, Elanor had a regular doctor and a regular place to go for health care, although she did not have health insurance from her job as a server in a local restaurant. Open about her sexuality, she usually disclosed her sexual identity to her health care providers and was out to family, friends, and co-workers.

The first time Elanor had sex it was with a man, and she was nineteen years old. She also had sex with a woman for the first time at nineteen. This was a common age among women in the study for initiation of sex, and for many women, first sex with women and first sex with men occurred within a close time period. Like many study participants, Elanor had never had a relationship with a man, but she had sex with men on occasion. With both men and women, Elanor tried to practice safer sex. For example, she always used condoms when having vaginal intercourse with a man, and with men, she sometimes also used condoms for oral sex. However, she rarely used a barrier (such as a latex dental dam) with women for oral sex because, she said, it was too much of a bother. Although she did wash sex toys, such as dildos, between partners, she also engaged in tribadism, or genital rubbing, with no barrier.

Elanor felt her HIV risk to be low, yet she was recently tested for HIV because she thought she was at risk. This reflects a common inconsistency in attitudes toward HIV among the women in this study. She usually dates straight or bisexual women, rather than women who identify as lesbian. Elanor says she uses alcohol in sexual situations because it makes it "much easier to be intimate."

Elanor's story embodies the confusion and many of the questions that are somewhat typical among women in this study. She exhibits some protective actions and some potentially risky actions. Yet she knows, from her own experience, there is a risk of woman-to-woman transmission. What factors prompt her action? Elanor is like many women in this study: aware of risk yet ambivalent about avoiding risk and utilizing protective actions. Some women do not know when or how to protect themselves. In fact, several women who volunteered for the study said they did so in order to get information on the subject. Many women who participated in this study asked us questions about safer sex for lesbians, about what activities potentially pose risks, and about what they could do to protect themselves. I offered all participants safer-sex kits, which included an STI leaflet from a lesbian health clinic, dental dams, lubricant, condoms, gloves, and finger cots.

Why are women so relatively uninformed? Until recently, most health issues, including HIV and STIs, have gone relatively unexamined among the lesbian population. Reasons for this research gap vary. The lesbian community is relatively hidden and therefore is not always readily accessible to researchers; general gender bias or sexism may play a role; or it may be that there is a lower incidence of HIV and STIs in this group, and higher-risk groups are more consistently brought to the attention of researchers. Lesbian health issues are now becoming a more popular focus of research. Nonetheless, knowledge regarding HIV and STIs among self-identified lesbian women is still incomplete.

Lesbians are often viewed in the academic and mainstream literature as unidimensional creatures whose lives revolve around their sexual orientation. The popular picture of a lesbian in the literature is that of a white, middle-class, educated, politically active or aware woman, with a high disposable income (Solarz, 1999). However, lesbians as a group are not homogenous, nor do they live in a vacuum, separate from other communities (Stevens, 1993). Lesbian women comprise a full spectrum of society. There are lesbians of color. There are lesbians who have sex with men. There are homeless lesbians, poor lesbians, rural lesbians, and injection-drug-using (IDU) lesbians (Lemp et al., 1995; Leifer and Young, 1997). Not to see the diversity among lesbians is itself a risk because if invisible, these subgroups are ignored by researchers, the health care industry, and society.

Are lesbians at risk for HIV and STIs? Opinions range from an emphatic "no" (Robertson and Schachter, 1981; Cohen et al., 1993; Raiteri, Fora, and Sinico, 1994), to "possibly" (Einhorn and Polgar, 1994), to "possibly, but not likely enough to merit extensive study" (Rothblum, 2000), to "yes" (Rankow, 1995; Morrow, 1996; Marrazzo, 2000a; Marrazzo, Koutsky, and Handsfield, 2001).

Sexual identity and sexual action are not synonymous. It is important to distinguish between identity and action, as it is not one's identity that puts one at risk but, one's actions (Fishbein and Guinan, 1996). Although the most common lesbian sexual acts may not in themselves put a woman at high risk for HIV or STIs, these are not the only factors involved. Knowing a partner's sexual history is important. Regardless of sexual identity, many HIV-positive women report having sex with other women (Bevier et al., 1995; Kennedy et al., 1995; Denenberg, 1997). Some women may contract HIV or a sexually transmitted infection before identifying as a lesbian, and others may hide an STI or even be unaware of having one (Hastie, 2000). A woman cannot evaluate a potential partner based on an identity label alone, neither can risk be narrowed to only sexual action. Instead, all risk factors should be explored (Shotsky, 1996).

Sexually transmitted infections and HIV have been reported in cases where self-reports of sexual contact are exclusively with other women (Tronosco et al., 1995; Solarz, 1999). However, STI and HIV risks for women who have sex with women (WSW) remain unclear. Although cases of woman-to-woman sexual transmission of HIV have been reported (Rochman, 1999), they have not yet been proven through virus matching. Studies indicate that STI transmission is more likely than HIV transmission. In fact, one group of researchers (Raiteri, Fora, and Sinico, 1994; Raiteri et al., 1998) tracked HIV-discordant couples an average of ten months and found no transmission. They concluded that the absence of "traumatic" sex, low-risk lesbian sexual practices, the low level of HIV in vaginal fluids, and a low rate of sex in lesbian couples all contributed to their findings. However, the study's conclusion of no risk was criticized for time frame, sample, and other methodological concerns (Reynolds, 1994). Also, focusing on couples rather than on single women, or both, will affect study results. Results from studies of STI transmission also conflict. For example, one study of bacterial vaginosis (McCaffrey et al., 1999) showed no woman-to-woman transmission, while others (Berger et al., 1995; Marble and Key, 1996) claim to confirm the woman-to-woman sexual transmission of bacterial vaginosis.

As a consequence of a growing body of research and rising awareness, guidelines for safer sex between women are becoming more available in places such as women's health clinics, AIDS organizations, and popular health books such as *The Lesbian Sex Book* (Caster, 1993) and *Making Out: The Book of Lesbian Sex and Sexuality* (Schramm-Evans, 1995). These books advocate safety measures when one is unsure of a partner's health status. Recommendations include the use of dental dams for oral sex, latex gloves for digital penetration, condoms on shared sex toys, and not sharing needles.

According to the Centers for Disease Control and Prevention (CDC) (1995), research does not reflect the information needed about risk and protective factors for women who have sex with women. This may be due to inconsistent terminology or to a divergence between sexual identity and action. Marginal populations are difficult to access, especially subgroups of racial and ethnic minorities and varied socioeconomic statuses. Woman-to-woman transmission of HIV and STIs is not well understood. The male-to-female transmission model may not apply. Drug abuse and sex with men are largely hidden actions within the lesbian community, so women may not know their partners' actual histories.

According to the Institute of Medicine (Solarz, 1999), in a recent comprehensive lesbian health report, the actual sex practices of women who have sex with women are unknown. Traditionally, the assumption was that there was no exchange of body fluids or contact between mucous membranes, implying that women who have sex with women were at low risk. More recent studies (Diamant, Lever, and Schuster, 2000; Morrow and Allsworth, 2000) show that the sexual practices of women who have sex with women often do involve exchange of body fluids and contact between mucous membranes. Transmission of some sexually transmitted infections, such as herpes, requires only skin contact. The CDC recommends further investigation into the actual sex practices of women who have sex with women, including sex during menstruation and the sharing of sex toys.

There have been few documented cases of woman-to-woman transmission of HIV, which may be due, in part, to cases being attributed to more traditionally accepted risk factors, such as illicit drug use or high-risk heterosexual actions (Kennedy et al., 1995). There seems to be a general belief not only in the lesbian community but also in the larger society that lesbians are protected from contraction of HIV or other STIs (Richters et al., 1998). This perception may lead women not to practice safer sex, such as using a barrier during oral sex. Unwillingness to disclose sexual identity and the lack of a need for birth control may lead lesbians to ignore their gynecological health (Eliason, 1996; Taylor, 1999), thus increasing the chances of HIV or an STI going undetected. In some cases, donor insemination may play a role (Centers for Disease Control and Prevention, 1999). In addition, lesbian women may know that safer sex can help protect them from transmission but, similar to heterosexual individuals, factors such as a sense of personal invulnerability (Yep, 1993) or low self-esteem (Cranston, 1992) may stop them from taking steps to protect themselves.

Although women may identify as lesbian, action and identity are sometimes divergent (Richters et al., 1998) and some women may exhibit bisexual actions while identifying as a lesbian (Kennedy et al., 1995; Eliason, 1996). In addition, definitions of *lesbian* and what constitutes "having sex" vary widely (Brogan et al., 2001). Identity-divergent action may occur in several contexts. For instance, women who are ambivalent about their sexual identity may engage in sexual activities with both men and women (Marrazzo, Koutsky, and Handsfield, 2001), and young lesbians have been found to be particularly vulnerable in this way (Pederson, 1994; Diamant et al., 1999). Other women who identify as lesbian may have potentially high-risk sex with men as a result of drugs or alcohol (Wilton, 1997). In that context, identity and action are incongruent, which may place a woman at higher risk, especially if she ignores the sexual actions with men. Other women have sex with men in exchange for money or drugs (Bevier et al., 1995) or for economic survival (Travers and Paoletti, 1999). Still others who identify as lesbian have sex with men because they enjoy it (Norman et al., 1996; Wilton, 1997). Some women identify as lesbian when partnered with women, and as bisexual when partnered with men. Unprotected sex with men may put not only these women at risk but potentially also their female partners. The CDC (1999) reported many HIV-positive women having sex with women (2,220 out of 109,311 HIV positive through 1998). However, information on women having sex with other women is missing for half of all cases.

The social and economic costs of the medical and health establishment's lack of attention to lesbian sexual health risks of transmission and detection are varied. Women who do not think they are at risk are less likely to practice protective actions (Eliason, 1996). The lack of education among health care and public health workers regarding risks for lesbians leads to a lack of knowledge and accessible information for lesbian women. Lesbian women often do not disclose their sexuality to their health care workers for fear of stigma or discrimination (Smith, Johnson, and Guenther, 1985; Rankow, 1995; Dean et al., 2000). These fears are based on both real experiences and imagined consequences. In addition, lesbian women may be less likely to have regular pap smears, and thus cervical cancer may go undetected (Solarz, 1999). Also, research has shown that human papilloma virus (HPV), which can lead to cervical cancer, is found in lesbians who have never had sex with men (Marrazzo, 2000a).

This study is an attempt to begin understanding the factors surrounding lesbian sexual heath and health care-seeking actions and to explore lesbian women's perceptions of susceptibility, risk, and protective actions.

The Institute of Medicine recently published *Lesbian Health: Current Assessment and Directions for the Future* (Solarz, 1999), which is the most comprehensive review to date of the information available regarding lesbian health and which contains a number of recommendations for research in the area.

The Institute of Medicine identified several research priorities:

- a better understanding of the actual health status of lesbian women;
- a more complete understanding of lesbian-specific health risks or protective factors;
- research attention to the possible impact of socioeconomic or cultural factors on lesbian health;
- better definitions of sexual orientation and the meaning of lesbian sexual orientation, with special attention to diversity within the lesbian population; and
- the identification of possible barriers to access to health care for lesbians.

In this study, I attempt to address several research gaps as outlined in the Institute of Medicine report. These include

- better understanding of the physical and mental health status of lesbian women;
- understanding risk factors and protective actions regarding lesbian health, particularly HIV and STI risks;
- understanding the conditions for which protective factors reduce risk;
- adding to the literature on the diversity of the lesbian population; and
- identifying possible barriers to health care.

I examine how lesbian women construct their health, and how identity, knowledge, and beliefs, through experience and interaction, shape constructions of risk and vulnerability. I explore the role of institutional neglect, on the part of researchers and the health care industry, with regard to risk normalization along with identity, social context, and social location. I address this problem using a combination of quantitative and qualitative data to examine constructions of risk perception, actual risk taking, and protective actions among lesbians, including their interpretations of these. I use quantitative data for descriptive analyses and qualitative data to generate explanatory models grounded in the data (Morse and Field, 1995).

This study grew out of my intersecting interests in HIV, STIs, and lesbian health while I was a faculty associate in the Rollins School of Public Health at Emory University. The Atlanta/Emory Center for AIDS Research (CFAR), located in the School of Public Health, requested proposals for developmental grants in underresearched areas of HIV/AIDS. The CDC had put out a meeting report (Centers for Disease Control and Prevention, 1995) detailing the research on lesbians and HIV risk and calling for new research in that area. My grant proposal was accepted for funding ($35,000), Institutional Review Board (IRB) approval was granted from Emory University, and research began in April 1998. The study design and methodology grew and changed throughout the year of research, with the resulting data being far more in depth and broad than I originally intended. The study design is an exploratory, qualitative project with a quantitative component designed to provide descriptive statistics.

RESEARCH METHODS

In developing my research questions, I used the following elements of the health belief model. Specifically, perceived susceptibility refers to the conceptions lesbians have regarding their risk of HIV or STI contraction. Perceived severity is one's level of knowledge regarding HIV and STIs. Perceived benefits of utilizing protective action (including obtaining health care) are relative to the cost. Barriers are those factors that serve as barriers to protection, including institutional and interpersonal factors. Cues to action are what actually prompt women to reduce risks and increase protective action. For example, in this study, contracting an STI led some women to initiate safer-sex practices. With regard to self-efficacy, to what extent do these women feel able to reduce risk and increase protective actions?

I also examined actual risk factors and protective actions, including sexual practices, what means (if any) are being used to protect against HIV and STIs, and what sort of health care these women are obtaining. In addition to the questions raised by the health belief model, I used the following as guiding questions in this research project: What information is available about HIV and sexually transmitted infections with regard to the lesbian community? What are the health care practices of lesbian women, specifically with regard to gynecological health, disclosure of sexuality to health care practitioners, and treatment by health care professionals? What role do alcohol or drugs play in sexual identity and risk actions?

SAMPLING

The target population for this study was lesbian women residing in a large southeastern city. To be eligible for participation in this study, women had to be at least eighteen years of age and self-select for participation as a lesbian. Self-identification was important so as not to impose the researchers' definitions on the subjects, but to allow their own definitions to emerge.

Lesbians remain a somewhat hidden population. Until a recent U.S. Supreme Court hearing, homosexual sex was illegal in many U.S. states, and individuals who practice it are generally stigmatized. The parameters of the population "lesbian" are unavailable, and thus a truly representative sample is not possible. However, I attempted sample diversity through recruiting participants at a wide range of places, including universities, a feminist bookstore, the Department of Family and Children's Services, a lesbian women's bar, women's organizations, and by word of mouth. I also recruited participants at the city's annual Gay Pride Festival, a three-day event attended by hundreds of thousands of people. I shared a festival booth with a women's health center and distributed safer-sex kits with a flier describing the study. The fliers stated that Emory University School of Public Health was conducting a study of HIV and sexually transmitted diseases among lesbians. The project was called the Lesbian Sex Project, and this was printed on the recruitment fliers, which asked that women over eighteen who were interested in participating in the study call the project phone number. The fliers also stated that there was a twenty-dollar payment for participation. The local southeast gay newspaper wrote an article about the study, which led a number of people to call and enroll. Contacts also included people who had been interviewed in a previous public health study and knew the researchers involved. The first women recruited were used as zero-stage respondents in the study. Zero-stage respondents are those who are the first in a social network to be recruited.

Snowball or chain-referral sampling was then used to expand the sample (Watters and Biernacki, 1989; Kaplan, Korf, and Sterk, 1987). The zero-stage respondents were asked to name women in their social network and to refer them to the study. Snowball sampling is effective in studying sensitive topics, as it can provide access to a hidden population. Sampling then proceeded from the zero-stage individuals who referred others they knew (first stage) and so on. Furthermore, as the data collection continued, theoretical sampling (Glaser and Strauss, 1967; Strauss and Corbin, 1990) was employed to ensure the inclusion of a wide variety of experiences.

Theoretical sampling is based on concepts that have "proven theoretical relevance" to the evolving theory. These concepts are significant by virtue of their being repeatedly present or absent when comparing incidents; and through coding, the concepts become categories. For example, one recurring concept in the study was the fear of disclosing one's sexual identity to health care workers. Categories and concepts evolve during grounded theory analysis, which begins with the first data collected (Glaser and Strauss, 1967; Strauss and Corbin, 1990). Theoretical sampling must be flexible; the researcher must be open to new relationships between data and new categories. Original sampling is open and narrows as concepts and theories emerge from the data. With theoretical sampling, theory is expanded by varying the sampling criteria and interview guide according to the current focus of analysis (Strauss and Corbin, 1990). For instance, in the present study, attempts were made to include women of different socioeconomic groups. In addition, when it was discovered that issues of sex work were often pertinent to the evolving analysis, the interview guide was altered to include more questions about those experiences and the attitudes and feelings regarding them.

DATA COLLECTION

After giving informed consent, all 162 participants completed the fifty-page survey, seventy completed the in-depth interviews (see the Appendix for the characteristics of the individual interviewees), and a different subsample of twenty-four women participated in a total of three focus groups. In-depth interview and focus-group participants were those who volunteered or were invited to participate after completing the survey. Since all six of the interviewers involved in this study were white middle-class females, it was especially important not to force our social constructs on women who might have had experiences that differed by ethnicity, race, or class (Krauss et al., 1997). Prior to participating, all women were informed in detail about the nature of the study and the content of the interview and were given an opportunity to ask questions. The participants were encouraged to ask questions and bring up other relevant information, and were informed that they did not have to answer any questions they did not want to answer. The interviews lasted between one and two hours. All but a few of the in-depth, qualitative interviews were audiotaped and transcribed as soon as possible after the interview. One interviewee refused to be taped, and two tapes were unintelligible. The interview recipients received twenty dollars for their time. No personal identifiers were included on any of the transcripts.

The survey element of the interview, in which all women participated, consisted of structured questions on demographic characteristics such as age, race, education, employment, sexual history, use of protection during sex, and drug and alcohol use history. Questions also included general knowledge of STIs and HIV, knowledge of risk factors regarding HIV and STIs, and knowledge of protective choices. Other questions concerned respondents' perceived risk, actual protective action, and attitudes toward lesbians and HIV and STIs. We also addressed health care-seeking action, disclosure of sexuality to health care professionals, and treatment by medical personnel.

We conducted three focus groups, one at the inception of the study, and the others staggered through the study. The purpose of the first focus group was to identify specific areas of concern and to get a general idea of what information was circulating in the lesbian community, and of where lesbians get their information about HIV and sexually transmitted infections. The first focus group was also used to aid in the development of specific questions for the in-depth interviews. The remaining focus groups were used to verify the information I was obtaining and to discuss preliminary findings and flesh out the quantitative data I was getting with narrative accounts. The focus groups and about two-thirds of the interviews took place in university offices. The remaining interviews took place in coffee shops, bookstores, a lesbian bar, and other on-campus locations.

DATA ANALYSIS

Qualitative data analysis was guided by grounded theory methodology (Glaser and Strauss, 1967; Strauss and Corbin, 1990). Using this methodology, data collection and analysis occur almost simultaneously, with the first focus group and the first few interviews being transcribed and coded immediately. The aim is to discover relevant social and social psychological factors as they emerge from the data and to modify interview questions and sampling procedures accordingly. Theoretical sampling, characteristic of grounded theory methodology, was employed throughout data collection in order to ensure a wide variety of responses, particularly with regard to race, age, and socioeconomic status.

After about the first five interviews were transcribed, I initiated open coding (Strauss and Corbin, 1990). I labeled the data according to content, using notes written in the margin. Concepts such as attitudes, events, and qualities were grouped under category labels. Each incident, idea, or event was given a name representing a phenomenon. These were based on what the phenomenon was or what it represented (i.e., properties of the phenomenon) (Strauss and Corbin, 1990). I examined each category and compared instances within categories using the constant comparison method, an integral component of grounded theory.

The constant comparison method consists of four stages (Glaser and Strauss, 1967). First, incidents within each category are compared. For example, one respondent described her feelings of shame about her STI and her lack of disclosure to partners. This incident was coded as belonging to the category of "barriers to safer sex" and was compared to other incidents within that category. The constant comparison begins to generate theories on the properties of the category. For instance, in this example, the element of shame was explored and compared to other barriers to safer sex, and types of stigma (shame about one's STI, embarrassment from one's partner potentially thinking one has an STI, and so on) were delineated. Next, categories and their properties are integrated. As the data collection and analysis simultaneously progressed, dozens of related subcategories were created, which were related to one another, and a list was compiled. I coded the remaining interview transcripts according to those categories, while the possibility of new emergent categories remained open. Incidents were compared with one another and with the accumulating emergent theory.

As more incidents were integrated into the theory, the theory broadened and fewer incidents required major modification in the theory as they fit into what has already been developed. At this stage, the theories began to solidify.

Another important component of the constant comparison method is theoretical saturation. As the data analysis progresses, the researcher examines each incident to see if it adds a new dimension to the theory. If no new dimensions are attained from repeated comparison of incidents, the category is said to be theoretically saturated, and researchers may modify the in-depth interview guides to explore new dimensions. Throughout this process, regular meetings and discussions were held by the research team on analytical, methodological, and theoretical issues. The use of grounded theory and the constant comparison method allows for the identification of relevant themes while maintaining individuals' stories. As the data collection continued, we were able to verify and challenge tentative findings with the aid of subsequent interviews and focus groups

Validity is a particular area of concern for qualitative research (Kirk and Miller, 1985). It is not always possible to discern whether the respondents are being truthful, and, just as important, whether the researcher is accurately portraying the respondents' points of view rather than imposing his or her own. In order to enhance the validity of this study, we employed several strategies. First, while obtaining informed consent from project participants, interviewers stressed how important it is to have accurate data. Because the study and its findings were personally relevant to respondents, they may have felt a personal investment in the outcome. That may increase the validity of the data. In addition, I used three data collection methods: a quantitative survey, qualitative interviews, and focus groups. This aided in verification of emergent themes. At least two members of the research team (I was one in every case) separately analyzed and coded interview and focus-group transcripts, and we discussed coding in staff meetings in order to enhance reliability and decrease subjectivity in analysis. The quantitative interview data, comprising 1,100 variables, were coded and entered into a statistical program, and double-checked for analysis. These data were used for descriptive statistics and exploration.

RESEARCH TEAM

Several people were involved in the design and implementation of this study. The two original research assistants on this project were both graduate students who identified as lesbian, one from the Department of Sociology and one from the Department of Women's Studies. They helped develop and pilot the interview guides. Later, three other lesbian women transcribed tapes and coded interviews. They were all sociologists who had some experience in public health.

DEFINITIONS OF TERMS

It is important to define our terms before beginning discussion.

lesbian: There is not one widely accepted definition of lesbian; definitions vary by study and by individual. Sexual orientation is most often described as including behavioral, affective (i.e., desire or attraction), and cognitive (i.e., identity) dimensions that occur across continua (Hunter, et al., 1998; Solarz, 1999). The Institute of Medicine, for example, focused on women who have sex with or primary emotional relationships with other women. For the purposes of the current study, *lesbian* is a self-identified category. This self-identification may be based on action, identity, and beliefs. Studies show that sexual identity labeling is not always congruent with action (e.g., a woman may call herself a lesbian but engage in occasional sex with men). Loosely, the definition of lesbian for this study is women who consider themselves to be lesbians; living women-centered lives; who are not heterosexual; who may or may not have sex with men or with women in the past, present, or in the perceived future; and who may or may not view lesbianism as a political issue.

protective actions: Actions, beliefs, and knowledge that protect one from exposure to or contraction of HIV or an STI. These may be the use of safer-sex materials (such as barriers), restricting sexual actions and partners, obtaining regular gynecological care, and being educated on the subject.

risk factors: Actions, beliefs, and knowledge that place one at risk for exposure to and possible contraction of HIV or an STI. These may include sex with a man, illicit drug use, sex work, and sex with a woman who has HIV or an STI.

LIMITATIONS OF STUDY

The results of this study are limited by several factors. The respondents all reside in the same southeastern city, so possible regional differences may not be reflected here, although some of the women were transplants to the area. Although targeted sampling was used to gather a representative sample, some subgroups are underrepresented or unintentionally left out. This study took place in a city that is very multiethnic. However, only English-speaking women were recruited for participation. Latina and Asian women especially were underrepresented. The definition of *lesbian* is hotly contested both within and without the lesbian community, and self-identification may have been affected by these debates. Also, a representative sample was not possible with a marginal, somewhat hidden population. The results of this study may not reflect everyone's definition of what it means to be a lesbian.

SAMPLE DESCRIPTION

The following are descriptive statistics on the 162 participants in the study. All 162 participants were female. They ranged in age from eighteen to fifty-five, with slightly more than half being in the twenty-six to thirty-five age group; 25 percent were between eighteen and twenty-five; the rest were over thirty-six. One of the goals of the study was the inclusion of nonwhite women. Sixty-seven percent of study participants were white, 26 percent black, and 7 percent other, mostly Latina, followed by Asian. These descriptive data are summarized in Table 1.1.

With regard to education, almost half of the sample had at least a college degree. Another 29 percent had some college, 27 percent had at least a high school diploma or a GED, and almost 6 percent had less than a high school degree. Most of the study participants (65 percent) worked full-time at the time of the study. Only 6 percent were full-time students. Respondents were asked to self-identify social class, and half identified as middle class. Thirty-eight percent identified as working class, about 10 percent as lower class or truly needy. Only 3 percent identified as upper class. I also asked respondents about their

TABLE 1.1. Characteristics of the Study Sample

Characteristic	Percentage (N)		Characteristic	Percentage (N)	
Age			*Race*		
18-25	25	(40)	White	67	(108)
26-35	54	(87)	Black	26	(42)
36-45	19	(31)	Other	7	(12)
46-55	2	(3)			
			Income		
Relationship status			$50,000+	8	(12)
Single	52	(84)	$40,000-$49,999	4	(6)
Same-sex nonresidential	19	(30)	$30,000-$39,999	16	(26)
Same-sex residential	25	(41)	$20,000-$29,999	24	(39)
Opposite sex	3	(5)	$10,000-$19,999	20	(32)
Other	1	(2)	<$10,000	28	(45)
Social class			*Education*		
Upper class	3	(5)	Less than HS	6	(9)
Middle class	50	(80)	HS or GED	17	(27)
Working class	38	(61)	Some college	29	(47)
Lower class	5	(9)	College degree	48	(79)
Truly needy	4	(6)			

Note: All respondents were female; N = 162. (Some section totals do not equal 162 due to missing data.)

individual income, and these results were spread widely. Twenty-eight percent of respondents reported less than $10,000 annual income. Some of these women were in relationships, however, in which their partners were the financial providers. Twenty percent of the women reported income between $10,000 and $20,000 a year, 24 percent between $20,000 and $30,000, 16 percent between $30,000 and $40,000, and 12 percent reported an annual income of more than $40,000.

More than half of the women were single at the time of the interview, 19 percent were in a nonresidential relationship with a same-sex partner, 25 percent lived with their same-sex partners, and 3 percent had an opposite-sex partner. Eighteen percent had children, most of whom proved to be from previous heterosexual relationships. A majority (64 percent) wanted children in the future.

BOOK ORGANIZATION

In Chapter 2, I describe the research literature and theoretical background of the study. The chapter contains a review of studies to-date on lesbians, HIV, and STIs. Social constructionism, symbolic interactionism, frame analysis, and the social psychology of health beliefs are discussed in relation to this study.

In Chapter 3, I discuss identity and the meaning of the labels that women in my sample selected to identify themselves. What do the words *lesbian, queer,* or *gay* mean to the people who choose them? On what basis are these labels chosen? The divergence between sexual identity and sexual action, as well as respondents' constructions of the meaning of their own sexual action and that of others, are also discussed in Chapter 4.

Risk and protective actions are the focus of Chapter 4. Descriptive statistics on the specific sexual activities of the women in the study, as well as their HIV and STI statuses are included. I examine how lesbian women's knowledge and beliefs contribute to their construction of susceptibility, risk, and protection.

In Chapter 5, I discuss risk from a public health standpoint and examine the protective actions individuals take. That discussion revolves around the use of barriers in sex, sexually transmitted infections, infidelity, HIV testing, sex with risky partners, needle sharing, and sex exchanges. In addition to constructions of risk, I address the women's justifications of risk-taking action.

Chapter 5 also includes a discussion of barriers to reducing risk. Women discussed drug and alcohol use, HIV knowledge, and myths and common perceptions of the lesbian community. They also face institutional barriers, such as the limited knowledge and unhelpful attitudes of many health care providers. I examine the women's reasons for not using protective actions, as well as their construction of beliefs and attitudes toward these barriers. I emphasize the importance of communication, feelings, and stigma. In addition, I examine cues to action. What are the perceived benefits of taking protective actions and reducing risk? What circumstances cue a woman to action? What plans do the women have for reducing sexually risky action in the future?

In Chapter 6, I discuss the ways in which this study contributes to the literature on lesbian sexual health. I review the implications of this study for public health, medicine, and sociology. I analyze the usefulness of the health belief model when applied to this population, and I note some methodological limitations and implications of this study.

Chapter 2

Background

LESBIAN WOMEN'S HEALTH ISSUES

Many major health risks associated with lesbian women are, of course, the same as those for heterosexual women, but there are some concerns specific to the lesbian population. The American Medical Association (AMA), in their recent policy on gay and lesbian health (Nation's Health, 1995) stated that sexual orientation should not be ignored. This contrasted with its 1981 policy, which addressed homosexuality with regard to only sexually transmitted infections and conversion to heterosexuality. According to a handbook on lesbian women's health (Wilton, 1997), several important factors distinguish lesbian health care from heterosexual women's health care. Among these factors are heterosexist health manuals, homophobia, and neglect by both medical research and health care providers. One population-based study (Diamant et al., 2000) found that lesbians were more likely than heterosexual women to drink heavily and less likely to be insured or to have regular pap smears.

Lesbian women also face other health risks. Many of these additional risks reflect their stigmatized social status, their sometimes limited access to health care, and health communication. These risks include cancer, family planning, mental health, substance abuse, violence, and sexual assault (Dean et al., 2000), along with a possibility of decreased societal and environmental resources (Saunders, 1999) as well as internalized homophobia (Williamson, 2000).

Lesbian women do test positive for STIs and HIV. Several researchers have examined the prevalence of STIs among lesbian women. Sexual transmission of hepatitis A was reported between lesbians with no other risk factors besides oral/genital and oral/anal contact (Walters and Rector, 1986). Edwards and Thin (1990) found a prevalence of sexually transmitted infections, including herpes (16 percent) and HPV (11 percent), among lesbians (defined by them as a woman in a relationship with another woman at the time of the study). Marrazzo (2000a) found HPV prevalent (30 percent) among women who have sex with women, and concluded that this virus is transmitted through woman-to-woman sexual activity. Diamant and colleagues (1999, 2000) found a 17 percent STI rate among lesbians polled through a national gay magazine. Morrow and Allsworth (2000) found that 24 percent of the lesbians and 38 percent of the bisexual women in their sample had a lifetime history of a sexually transmitted infection. Their sample was recruited at women's events, health clinics, and HIV or STI clinics.

HIV research has tended to focus on what the CDC has defined as the major risk groups. These include IDUs, men who have sex with men (MSM), and sexual partners of people in those groups. In fact, for half of the women testing positive for HIV, no information was collected on whether they had had sex with another woman (Centers for Disease Control and Prevention, 1997). Research that does address lesbian women focuses on those women who report having sex with another woman within a specified period of time, usually three months. These studies most often concentrate on women who report other acknowledged HIV risks, such as injection-drug use. Women who have sex primarily or exclusively with women have been ignored as a risk group. The CDC reports that information is routinely obtained on AIDS cases among WSWs (Centers for Disease Control and Prevention, 1999). However, these women are not viewed as a risk category. In a recent report, about 22 percent of the female AIDS cases in Georgia fell under the category "risk not reported/other" (Georgia Department of Human Resources, 2001). Although some WSWs may be counted here, others are counted under different risk categories, such as sex with men or injection-drug use.

Young, Weissman, and Cohen (1992) reported that strategies to aid in intervention and prevention efforts among WSWs were scant because basic HIV research does not adequately address the needs of these women. An Italian research group (Raiteri et al., 1994) tested 181 lesbians for HIV and found eleven positive. Of those, ten were also IDUs. They also found that other sexually transmitted infections were more common in this group of women who injected drugs. They concluded that intervention and prevention efforts aimed at WSWs for HIV and STIs were far from adequate. Not one of the 181 women in their sample reported using protection during homosexual sex.

Stevens (1994a), conducted a study of HIV-risk practices of lesbian and bisexual women, interviewing 626 women recruited at women's bars. She found that there was a cultural construction of safety from HIV among WSWs, that WSWs inconsistently practiced safer sex, and that there was a lack of awareness among WSWs as to possible risk of HIV. Perry (1994, 1995), using the health belief model to examine 152 self-identified lesbian and bisexual white, middle class, college-educated women, found that WSWs were engaging in potentially high-risk sexual activities, such as performing oral sex on a menstruating partner, and showed little awareness of that risk. In addition, those with increased perceived susceptibility were more likely to use barrier methods of protection.

The literature (Stevens, 1994a; Perry, 1995) also points to the role of alcohol and other drugs in HIV- and STI-risk action among lesbians. Those who reported more frequent drinking were more likely to have sex outside their primary relationship and more likely to have anonymous sex. Others (Leigh and Stall, 1993; Young et al., 2000) also found that alcohol and drugs, including injection drugs, play a role in the sexual risk-taking action of WSWs. Lesbians who rely on the bar scene for social interaction used alcohol more than others (Heffernan, 1998). Other areas of concern are a lack of STI detection (as a factor in transmitting infections) and depression as related to risky sexual actions (White and Levinson, 1995).

Lemp and colleagues (1995) reported a high incidence of injection-drug use (4 percent), unprotected sex with women (92 percent) and sex with men (73 percent; of those, 40 percent had unprotected sex) among WSWs. Deren and colleagues (1999) examined the relative risks of injection-drug use and unprotected sex for HIV contraction among male and female IDUs and found that risks from sex-related actions were greater than risks from drug-related actions for the men and the bisexual women. Their results indicate that HIV-prevention efforts targeting homosexual and bisexual injection-drug users should be more focused on sexual actions than on traditional IDU-prevention strategies, which tend to focus on drug use alone.

Their findings strongly indicate the need for more research in this area.

A study by Kral and colleagues (1997) regarding the HIV risks of women who inject drugs (N = 3,856) included a subset of 231 women who reported having had sex with another woman in the thirty days prior to the interview. Only 6 percent of those women reported using barrier protection while giving oral sex, and only 3 percent while receiving it. Fifty percent of those WSWs also reported having had sex with a man during that time period. Magura, O'Day, and Rosenblum (1992) have shown that female IDUs who are also sexual partners are more likely to share needles that are not cleaned, due to the intimacy of their relationship.

Other recent research on sexual identity and HIV and STI risk among lesbians indicates that there are several risk factors that should be explored in depth. One is the likelihood that younger WSWs experiment sexually with men more than older WSWs (Diamant et al., 1999), and that often this experimentation is carried out with male friends who have sex with men, a major risk group for HIV (Cochran and Mays, 1996). In a survey of 350 WSWs, Cochran found that 26 percent reported sex with a man in the past year, and 19 percent reported sex with an MSM in the three months prior to the interview. In addition, the study results showed that African-American WSWs were more likely than white WSWs to be heterosexually active.

Maguen and Armistead (2000) examined the prevalence of unprotected sex among lesbian youth in the U.S. South and found that while fewer than one-half of their respondents had been tested for HIV, most reported risky sexual actions. They found that those who had been tested for HIV were much more aware of risk and protective factors and were more likely to utilize that knowledge. Adding to the area of risk actions, Fethers and colleagues (2000) examined medical records of women attending a public STI/HIV clinic in Australia between 1991 and 1998 and compared women who reported having sex with women to those who had not. They found a higher prevalence of bacterial vaginosis, hepatitis C, and increased HIV-risk actions among WSWs.

Myer (1997) used the health belief model to analyze lesbians' beliefs and practices surrounding HIV. The sample was somewhat homogeneous, representing educated, white, middle-class women. Among the 248 women who responded to the survey, most participated in some actions which could potentially place them at risk for HIV or STI transmission, including performing oral sex on a menstruating partner. Kahala (1999) also used the health belief model, conducting five in-depth interviews with lesbian women about their feelings regarding HIV risk. She found that her respondents maintained a conviction of safety and felt they were not at risk. They either denied their own risk or intuitively felt safe. Kahala found that, contrary to the health belief model, which postulates that knowledge of a risk reduces risk action, the women in her study were aware of risks but did not feel personally susceptible or reduce risk actions.

In their literature review, the Institute of Medicine delineates several frameworks for looking at lesbian health. The first is the larger context in which health actions take place. They suggest taking societal factors into account, such as possible stigma and discrimination due to sexual orientation or race. Researchers should examine other possible structural, financial, personal, and cultural barriers to avoiding risk or taking preventive health-related measures. Also, the role of the health care system and the attitudes of health care workers toward homosexuality may be a factor in health action decisions. These issues may include difficulty in finding lesbian-friendly health care providers, lack of household health insurance, and difficulty in communicating actual actions to health care providers due to perceived (or actual) homophobia (Solarz, 1999).

The literature suggests that although lesbian women are, to a large degree, knowledgeable about sexual health risks, they are still engaging in risk actions and failing to utilize protective strategies. This leads to the question of *why?* The current study seeks to answer that question.

Studies about lesbians and STI and HIV transmission have been limited by a number of factors (Centers for Disease Control and Prevention, 1999; Solarz, 1999; Dean et al., 2000; Brogan et al., 2001). These include inconsistencies in the definitions of sexual orientation, a lack of standard measures in this area, and a lack of control groups. In addition, lesbians are not readily identifiable, therefore the samples tend to overrepresent white, middle class, educated women who are available through university or lesbian-specific settings such as bars or activist groups. This skews samples. The available literature also tends to be very quantitative and reductive. It can be limiting to use strictly quantitative methods in an area in which knowledge is sketchy (Kirk and Miller, 1985).

Other researchers recommend targeted sampling of racial and ethnic groups, varied socioeconomic classes, ages, religious affiliations, and geographic locations. The Institute of Medicine (Solarz, 1999) also recommends snowball sampling and combined strategies to examine lesbian health. This study attempts to address these factors in sampling and interview question development, and also by examining drug and alcohol use, sexual actions with men, and sex work. This study provides additional needed data on risk and protective factors in this population.

THEORETICAL FRAMEWORK

In this study I used symbolic interaction and critical social constructionism to formulate questions, to guide the study, and to analyze data. Constructionist theory seeks to understand how people view their own world (Henry, 2001), rather than relying on some objective definition of reality. According to this perspective, reality is socially constructed. Factors such as identity, knowledge, and beliefs, informed by cultural and subcultural affiliations, form perceptions of reality and can lead individuals to have different interpretations of the same facts. These factors were taken into account in the research design, implementation, and analysis. Thus, the respondents in this study identified many of the relevant themes.

Individuals tend to take many aspects of their social realities for granted (Berger and Luckman, 1967). Once a definition of an experience or phenomenon is set, it can remain the accepted definition, regardless of the "objective facts" of the situation. For example lesbians are not generally believed to be at risk for HIV or STI contraction. This perception endures despite a growing body of literature to the contrary. Context is an important factor in the construction of reality (Berger and Luckman, 1967). An objective set of facts will take on different meaning according to context. Before an individual enters a social group or particular context, shared perceptions and knowledge already exist for that group (Berger and Luckman, 1967). When an individual becomes part of a group, she or he most likely accepts the preexisting knowledge and perceptions of that group as natural and real. So when a woman becomes part of a lesbian community, she is likely to take on the accepted knowledge of that community regarding HIV and sexually transmitted infections. Knowledge guides people's conduct in everyday life. This includes sexual conduct and sexual-risk-taking actions. People enter different social contexts with an idea of how to behave based both on experience and on shared knowledge.

According to Schutz (1962) and Berger and Luckman (1967), a social stock of knowledge exists for a given situation. Furthermore, use of this stock of knowledge allows individuals to assume with whom they are interacting and how they interact. Thus, in the context of a woman-to-woman sexual encounter, an individual might locate her partner as a lesbian and, based on the community-held belief that lesbians are not susceptible to sexually transmitting infections, make the assumption that the partner does not pose a health risk.

People act in relation to a set of meanings that are socially constructed (Waters, 1994). A key tenet of symbolic interactionism is that individuals act toward things (institutions, values, situations, people) on the basis of the meaning these things have for them (Blumer, 1969). These meanings, or knowledge, arise from social interactions and experience. Worldview, identity, and beliefs are constructed by social interaction through symbols, myths, institutions, and norms.

In addition to the stigma that comes with homosexuality, having a sexually transmitted infection can be stigmatizing as well. Goffman (1963) notes the importance of stigma management and spoiled identities. Goffman discusses three types of stigma: physical deformities, mental disorders, and "tribal" stigma. Tribal stigma comes from larger group membership, such as race or nation. As a discredited individual with a spoiled identity, the stigmatized person will try to manage information about the stigmatizing attribute. For example, a woman will control who has information about her sexually transmitted infection.

The principle of symbolization (Snow, 2001) focuses on the ways that objects and phenomena take on particular meanings. The traditional symbolic interactionist view holds that individuals are constantly interpreting the world around them. The principal of symbolization helps to uncover how often meanings come to individuals through an existing cultural condition (Snow, 2001). Goffman (1974) developed a schema of interpretive frameworks that contain or inhibit meaning. These frames are not individual constructions, rather, they exist at the level of the group, where they are often taken for granted. These frames are not unchanging. They also do not necessarily work for every situation in which one finds oneself (Snow, 2001). Goffman's primary social frameworks provide background understanding. The frame one engages in any situation provides a way of explaining the situation.

Symbolic interactionism and social constructionism provide the analytic tools to examine an individual's own definitions of risk, and to locate those definitions within the context of lesbian communities as well as within the surrounding culture. In addition, these frameworks undergird an analytic approach called the health belief model.

The health belief model (HBM) was developed in the 1950s by a group of social scientists to address public health issues from a social psychological perspective (Kiser, 1990). It was originally designed to determine why individuals failed to participate in illness-prevention or -detection programs (Glanz, Lewis, and Rimer, 1997). It was later extended to examine the relationship between behavior, illness, and health-related actions. It has been used to study HIV risks and protective actions among women with multiple risk actions (Gielen et al., 1994), among African-American subgroups (Cochran and Mays, 1993), and within multicultural groups in Asia (Quah, 1998). The model concerns how an individual constructs health beliefs surrounding risk and protective actions with regard to health threats. The main concepts of the HBM include perceived susceptibility, perceived severity, perceived benefits, perceived barriers, cues to action, and self-efficacy. The HBM views health actions from the subjective perspective of the actor (Whetsell, 1990).

Perceptions of susceptibility refer to whether an individual thinks he or she will contract an infection. Perceived susceptibility is influenced by sociological, demographic, and structural factors (Kiser, 1990). Research shows that the perceived susceptibility of lesbians to both HIV and sexually transmitted infections is generally low and may be due to a lack of data and knowledge, a dearth of open discussion, unwillingness to change conceptions, misinformation, and being closeted with health care professionals.

Perceived benefits refer to whether the individual feels that the action or preventive action will have benefits that outweigh the perceived costs. In other words, is the benefit of avoiding risk and utilizing protective actions greater than the potential cost? Perceived barriers include feeling unable to perform the beneficial action for various reasons, such as having one's judgment clouded by alcohol or drugs, a lack of control over safer sex practices, unwillingness to practice safer sex actions, sexual identity issues, and apathy. Perceived barriers may be institutional, such as sexism, heterosexism, and homophobia (Grossman, 1994; Eliason, 1996; Williamson, 2000). Barriers are also perceived differently under different circumstances (Fishbein and Guinan, 1996).

Cues to action refer to the factors that impel individuals to practice preventive actions or reduce risk. When are these factors relevant? In what situations? These cues to action may include education, personal experiences, or beliefs (Kiser, 1990). Self-efficacy is a person's belief in his or her ability to make positive choices.

According to the HBM, if an individual perceives a threat and sees it as personally relevant and preventable, he or she will take action to thwart the threat. However, that is not always what happens. Modifying factors such as age, sex, and so on affect how people view their susceptibility. Components of the HBM (Strecher and Rosenstock, 1997) were used in this study. Although the HBM is generally used quantitatively, some studies have used it in qualitative exploratory studies, as quantitative data often fail to provide context (Whetsell, 1990). This study employs the HBM framework to form both quantitative and qualitative research questions and to guide the analysis of the qualitative data by providing preliminary categories for coding used in the grounded theory analysis. From these preliminary categories, respondents' experiences and stories were analyzed in the context of symbolic interactionism and social constructionist theories. In addition, Goffman's (1974) concept of interpretive frameworks was applied.

Sexual identity is a critical concept in this study. How does one take on a lesbian identity? Many factors influence an individual's decision to internalize an identity and to disclose that identity to others. These include a larger culture of homophobia, heterosexual socialization, and individual factors (Eliason, 1996). Some research has focused on developmental models of coming out. Cass (1996) developed a psychosocial model called sexual identity formation, which integrates both psychological and social factors. Three factors comprise this model: (1) perception of oneself as being lesbian, (2) perceptions of one's behavior as being lesbian, and (3) others' perceptions of the individual's sexual identity.

Sexual identity formation and negotiation are more fluid among lesbians than among gay men (Hunter et al., 1998). Troiden (1989) found that women's sexual identity formation was not necessarily one-way; it may change over time as women move between identifying or acting as lesbian, bisexual, and even straight. Bisexual identity formation is not clear-cut either, as there are no clear communities or guidelines (Hunter et al., 1998), and this can be a barrier to disclosing one's bisexual status. In addition, Hunter and colleagues (1998) point out that sexual identity formation and disclosure are not uniform across cultures or cultural subgroups.

Most models of sexual identity formation examine changes through stages (Cass, 1996; Faderman, 1984; Troiden, 1989). Sexual identity is often viewed as a self-labeling process, without great attention to outside factors such as social interaction and interpersonal relations (Cox and Gallois, 1996). Social identity theory examines the process of identity in addition to self-labeling. According to this perspective, sexual identity is not static, and it is influenced not only by perceptions of self but also by perceptions of others in an individual's reference groups; from other, indirect sources of information derived from the larger culture; and from the intersection of an individual's other identities (Cox and Gallois, 1996).

Chapter 3

Issues of Identity and Action

Shawn was a twenty-nine-year-old African-American woman who had some college experience and worked full-time. She earned $25,000 to $30,000 a year and considered herself to be working-class. She lived with her female partner, with whom she raised two children (both from her partner's previous relationship). Although Shawn had never been pregnant, she planned to get pregnant one day through an at-home insemination, meaning in her case that she will not have sex with a man; rather, she (or her partner) will inseminate herself with a friend's sperm.

Shawn was in very good health, had a regular doctor, and had health insurance for the six months prior to the interview. She said she always disclosed her sexual identity (lesbian) to her health care professionals, as well as to her family, friends, and co-workers. Shawn had never had a sexually transmitted infection. She had never had sex with a man and said she is very likely to ask female partners about sexually transmitted infections and HIV. Shawn first had sex with a woman at age fifteen. As far as protective factors, she always used condoms on sex toys when sharing with partners, and always changed the condom between partners, but rarely used dental dams or similar barriers for oral sex. She had performed oral sex on a menstruating partner, and had never used barrier protection when doing so, she said, "Because I felt comfortable with the person. I had been around them for X amount of time, so that's why I didn't use it." She also engaged in genital rubbing and in anal rimming with no barrier. She said she did not use protection because she trusted her partner and, to her knowledge, she had never had a partner with a sexually transmitted infection. Shawn had tried crack cocaine and marijuana and was a regular drinker (sixteen to twenty days per month). Although Shawn considered herself at low risk for HIV, she had been tested ten times, at testing sites and in jail. She felt she was at low risk because she always used condoms and dental dams with casual partners who, in her view, were the potentially dangerous partners.

Shawn felt that the lesbian community "is all about status." She said she will call herself a lesbian but prefers the term "stud." Shawn spent time in jail, where she had a romantic and sexual relationship with a cellmate. One time she was in love with a woman who steadfastly refused to have sex with her, and finally told her it was because she was HIV positive. Even though Shawn identified as lesbian and had never had sex with a man, she pointed out that she had almost been at risk for HIV with this woman she had been in love with who was positive. Shawn was quite clear in her sexual identity, and had been since an early age. She had always known she was a lesbian, and had never been interested in sexually experimenting with men.

IDENTITY LABELS

For some women, sexual identity is not as cut-and-dried as it was for Shawn. The women in this study were asked, "How would you classify your current sexual identity?" The question referred to a particular point in time, that of the interview. Sexual identity classification can change over time, and one's sexual identity label may not always match one's sexual actions. Table 3.1 shows label choices for this sample.

For the women I surveyed, the choice of a label for their sexual identity varied widely. Most respondents (62 percent) chose to identify as *lesbian*. Another 9 percent preferred the term *gay*, and 7 percent *queer*. A little more than 15 percent classified themselves as *bisexual* and 3 percent said they are currently straight. Those women who classified themselves as straight have or have had sexual and romantic primary relationships with women, and self-selected to participate based on study criteria. Almost 4 percent chose "other" and wrote in *dyke* or *transgendered*. The person who wrote in *transgendered* was the only person to bring up that term. Richters and colleagues (1998) found that those women who identified as trans-

TABLE 3.1. Sexual Identity Labels

Label	Percentage	N
Lesbian	62	101
Bisexual	15	25
Gay	9	15
Queer	7	11
Other (including, written in, "dyke" and "transgendered")	4	6
Straight	3	4

gendered were more likely to choose *other* than *lesbian* as a category. I did not think to include any questions on gender identity in our questionnaire, and I will include them in future studies on sexual identity. The breakdown of label choices is close to findings from similar studies, although each study had a different method of recruiting and a different way of defining *lesbian.*

Recruitment of lesbians for research studies has typically been through self-identification. Many researchers recruit participants through specifically gay sources, such as festivals, bookstores, and magazines, where one would expect to find self-identified lesbians. Richters and colleagues (1998) recruited 585 women at a gay festival. Of those, 58 percent identified as lesbian or homosexual, 15 percent as bisexual, and 5 percent as straight. Morrow and Allsworth (2000) found that 87 percent of their sample (N = 504) identified as lesbian and 13 percent as bisexual. There are no uniform measures for defining lesbians. Brogan and colleagues (2001) suggest that sexual identity should be measured by both self-identification and actions in order to evaluate health risks. Later in this chapter I discuss how identity and actions are not always congruent, and how these differing meanings may lead women to minimize protective actions.

Sexual identity is comprised of several elements; it is not just with whom one prefers to have sex. These elements include (but are not limited to) one's biological sex; the biological sex of one's partner; one's assigned gender; one's gender identity; one's political identity; one's partner preference (sexual and emotional); and one's sexual actions. The elements that are important in choosing one's label and the degree to which they are deemed important vary.

BASIS OF LABEL CHOICE

Sexual identity labeling is subjective; even for women in the same circumstances with similar descriptions, label choice is not uniform. For example, one respondent said that although both she and her female partner had been sexually involved with men in the past, their self-identification differs. She said,

> My girlfriend identifies as gay, even though she's also had male partners. I identify as bisexual because I have been in love with a

man—one man—so I feel like I still have the potential to be in love with a man again in my life, therefore I identify as bisexual.

In this woman's case, it was not just who her current partner was, or what her current identity was; rather, her identity labeling included past and potential love interests. Although their actions were similar, their self-identification differed.

Individual women's definitions are not the only ones lacking uniformity. Researchers also have not tended to use standard definitions for sexual identity. Studies by the CDC and others focused on actions as they defined lesbians as women who, since 1977, have had sex exclusively with women (Stevens, 1993). Others base their definition on attraction and define a lesbian as "a woman who is primarily physically and emotionally attracted to women" (Diamant et al., 1999, p. 98). The most encompassing basis of label choice for women in my sample was preference. For some, it was simply a matter of with whom they had sex. As one woman put it, "I identify as bisexual because I mess with both sexes." Another defined lesbian as "a biological woman who is attracted to other women." For many others, it was a more complex matter of preference. One woman defined her self-label, *dyke,* as "Steadfastness, I don't know, just an individual, strong, self-supporting woman, you know, who prefers to go to bed with women." Definitions included emotional attachments, in that label choice was related to whom one loved. One woman articulated a common theme in this way:

> Someone who exclusively likes to be with women, sexually and emotionally wants to spend their lives with another woman. Or maybe they just have that kind of identity; they may be celibate their whole life, but their identity is lesbian, or women-focused.

This respondent incorporated women who were not sexually active into her definition. Many people define sexual identity in general on the basis of sexual actions alone, and that definition ignores those who may be celibate for periods of time, or for their entire lifetime.

For some lesbians, labeling is a matter of political preference and the choice to be in the group "lesbians." This is related to notions of unity and separateness. Annette, a twenty-seven-year-old white woman who identified herself as "queer," described it this way:

I guess being queer means that you—you are kind of separate from a lot of mainstream values. But at the same time I guess I choose the term *queer* because I kind of feel separate from some lesbian or gay values, too. I think being queer gives you a lot more space to be yourself than a lot of people who have rigid roles laid out for them.

For Annette, the choice of *queer* distinguished her from both mainstream and lesbian values. The terms *lesbian* and *straight* felt too restrictive to her. Michelle, a twenty-four-year-old white, single female who identifies as gay, wanted to feel connected to a queer community:

INTERVIEWER: So how did you say—what word did you say you use to define your sexual identity?

MICHELLE: I think I said *gay,* actually. Yeah, I did. I say—I guess I say *gay* more than anything else. Like if someone says, like I would say in conversation, "I'm gay," is probably what I say more than anything. I don't say bisexual anymore, even though I did when I first came out. I mean, I think lots of people do when they first come out, because it is too scary. And I don't think that my sexual behavior or my orientation have changed any since then, but I think I just felt less comfortable bisexual because I felt more like I wanted to identify with a queer community, and bisexual is not socially acceptable in a lot of parts of queer communities. And also just because I wanted to be sort of unequivocally identified with gay people, or with a lesbian community.

Michelle's statement illustrates the perception of bisexuality as both a transition and a stigmatized status. Her sexual behavior had not changed, but her label had. For Michelle, the choice of label was a conscious one, and it was not based entirely on her behavior. Nor was the choice of Tawna, a twenty-nine-year-old, single, African-American woman who described herself as a lesbian-identified bisexual:

Because I'm one of those feminist people that thinks that my lesbian identity is about my politics. And also, I don't want to minimize my attraction to women. I have a different kind of attraction to women. When I'm with a woman, it's more passionate, more profound. I feel more connected.

Tawna emphasized the political aspect of her identity and her attraction to women while also acknowledging her bisexual actions. For Tawna, it was a combination of politics and emotions. For others, it may be a combination of emotions and tactile preferences. One focus-group participant described it this way:

> Well, I like sex with men, but I don't like cuddling men. That's my problem. That's why I prefer women. I don't like the way [men] smell very much, and I really don't like their texture. And that's why I don't want to roll over in the middle of the night and say, "Gosh, I wish I could make him come again." With women I do.

For this woman, it was a matter of choice based on desire and preference. In addition to politics, emotions, and preferences, stereotypes, a lack (or presence) of rigid roles, and other people's definitions and reactions also play a part in label choice. Stigma and internalized homophobia led one woman to call herself straight although she had had sex and emotional relationships with women all of her adult life. She said she defined a lesbian as a "big, fat, ugly bulldyke," and while she said her girlfriend was a lesbian according to her definition, she did not feel that this label fit her. She admitted to being extremely homophobic and called it "total dissociation." This dissociation between identity and action could potentially lead to self-homophobia.

Often, lesbian women will have a strong opinion of what it means to be a lesbian. One woman related how her identity had been questioned by both heterosexuals and lesbians, who had said, " 'You're not a very good lesbian,' because I don't fit the standard definition of 'I hate men' and I don't only want to fuck women and whatever. I don't fit that." This comment reflects some of the discord even within the lesbian community about what it means to be a real lesbian. Critics include so-called "gold-star" lesbians (those who have never had sex with a man), and sometimes members of this group stigmatize women who currently choose or have chosen in the past to be sexually active with men.

Sexual identity labeling is not static. It can change over time and also by circumstance. One's self-label may change with the gender of one's partner or by changing life goals. One woman said she describes herself as dyke when she is involved with a woman, as bisexual when she is involved with a man, and queer as an overriding label. For her, labeling is situational, but some women eschew labels altogether. One woman said that if she had to label herself, "I guess I would say I'm a deitistic Christian, SM, leather, Latina dyke who is transgendered." These women paint a complex picture of what sexual identity means and what bases are used in deciding how to identify. It is clear, however, that sexual identity and sexual actions are not always congruent.

IDENTITY AND SEXUAL ACTION

Lorna had identified as a lesbian since she was nineteen years old. She was a thirty-three-year-old white woman with a high school degree. At the time of the study she was unemployed, making less than $10,000 in the prior year. She said she considered herself to be working class, and was living with her female partner. Lorna said she was in excellent health and, although she was HIV positive, wanted to be pregnant again someday. This time, she said, she will go to a clinic for insemination. She had Medicaid and regularly visited a community clinic for health care. Unlike most other women in the study, Lorna said her sexual identity was a conscious choice:

INTERVIEWER: At what point did you identify as a lesbian?

LORNA: I guess when I was about nineteen. I was real close to this person and it just happened. And I was like that anyway—I had had my share of guys and I had some real bad experiences with them, so I decided to go to the other side. And so that's where I've been for thirteen or fourteen years.

INTERVIEWER: So it was a conscious choice then?

LORNA: Yes.

While several women discussed the divergence of identity and action, Lorna was the only participant who said her sexual identity was completely a choice. Like many women in the sample, she had had sex with men, but had never had a relationship with one. Lorna first had sex when she was eighteen years old, with a man, and she was nineteen years old when she first had sex with a woman. She decided at that time that she was a lesbian. One sexual encounter, in which she was trying to get pregnant, left her HIV positive. Her current female partner is also HIV positive and they met at a local shelter for women with HIV. Lorna said she is more comfortable with a partner who is also HIV positive because she does not have to worry about constantly disclosing her status or about taking precautions for every sexual activity.

Lorna said she always uses protection during sex because, as she said, "I don't need anything on top of this [HIV]." However, when asked about individual sexual encounters, she recalled not using protection on many occasions. She had two children, one of whom was born after her HIV transmission (at the time of the study, that child was testing negative for HIV).

Although Lorna had only had sex with women in the year prior to the interview, she was treated for a new trichomoniasis infection in that time period. Although Lorna said she always used condoms when she had sex with men, she did not use a condom the last time she had sex with a man. However, she said she consistently used dental dams when having oral sex with a woman, or when a woman was having oral sex with her, including when either partner was menstruating. Lorna also engaged in tribadism (genital-to-genital rubbing) without barrier protection, but she used barriers when anal rimming. When sharing dildos, she said she was sure to wash them between partners. She had never exchanged sex for money or goods. She had smoked crack, but said she did not drink. She had one HIV test, and that was because she thought she was at risk. That test came back positive. Lorna described how this result changed her life:

INTERVIEWER: What's the biggest change that your life has taken?

LORNA: I have to take medicine. I have to go to the clinic and people are like, "Oooh, does she have the total package?" But that's the biggest change—I have to take medicine. Other than that I do everything that I was normally doing. I have to be cautious sometimes. You know, when it's that time of the month around my kids. I have to be careful that I don't cut my hand by accident when my kids are near and they have scratches and I touch them. I have to be really cautious and I live it every day so I am used to it.

Lorna's sexual actions are similar to those of many women in this study. She had had sex with both men and women, but identified as a lesbian and preferred to have sex only with women. Most study participants first had sex in their late teens (80 percent) and about 10 percent first had sex in their twenties. Nearly 10 percent first had sex before they were ten years old, indicating, in many cases, sexual abuse. One young woman had not yet had sex at all. Of those women who have had sex with men, the majority said that it occurred in their teens. The same is true for first sex with women, but a significant number indicated that their first sexual encounter with a woman was while they were in their twenties.

Identity labels do not always directly correspond with preferences for sex partner (Centers for Disease Control and Prevention, 1999). Einhorn and Polgar (1994) found that only 47 percent of those women who identified as lesbian have had sex exclusively with women since 1978 (for bisexual women, it was ten percent). First of all, there is no clear consensus on what the labels mean, or who gets to define them. Also, what constitutes the act of sex is unclear and debatable and is especially muddy when discussing lesbian sex. Also, labels are fluid, and definitions are subjective. When a woman has sex with both men and women and identifies as bisexual, it is easy to understand. When a woman identifies as lesbian, gay, queer, or homosexual and has sex with men, it is less clear. There are many reasons why lesbians have sex with men. Abigail, a forty-five-year-old white woman with genital herpes who had not had sex with a man in the past year, described the changes her sexual identity has taken over the years:

Okay. Um, I think, well, I was a tomboy, and I wasn't particularly concerned about my sexual identity. But I was, I was different from my friends in high school, in that—I mean I went out with men and I had sex with men, but they were more interested in men than I was. And if I had the vocabulary at the time, which I didn't, I would have said I was bisexual. Which I am probably bisexual. I mean I am bisexual so far as enjoying sex with men or women. So, um, I only dated men and had sex with men up until about I was twenty-one. [Before then she only had sex with men, not women.] But I had, I had feelings of attraction for women throughout my adolescence and life, sort of. I was attracted to everybody, it didn't matter [laughs]. So, but I didn't think in terms of bisexual or lesbian or heterosexual or anything like that, since nobody really talked about it, it seems like then. So, I fell in love with a man when I was like nineteen years old, and we were together for like five years. And I was also attracted to women during that time. And we were both, um, alcoholic and drug addicts. I was—I had—um, I was an alcoholic and drug addict from a very early age, like thirteen, then I went to treatment at about twenty-six. So all of that with him was during the time before I got sober. I don't know how old I was, early twenties, when I started—he was actually in jail—and I started acting on my feelings for women. And, um, it was like seventy, midseventies. So I, um, discovered feminism, which enlightened me in many spheres. And I realized that I just felt identified, I felt that I identified as a lesbian. Because I read some lesbian feminist literature and it made a lot of sense to me. It was things I already knew, but it was being articulated. So, after, after that point in the midseventies, I thought of myself as a lesbian and only had relationships with women. Until I went to treatment, got sober and was not—didn't have really, I had short-term relationships with women as I was recovering, I would say. Then as I got more well, emotionally and every other way, I started having more substantial relationships [with women].

Abigail's changes in her self-identity label came along with changes in her life and in how she viewed herself. Age, feminism, and education all played roles in her identity development. For other women, the label of lesbian is simply a matter of comfort. They may have a bisexual identity and attraction, but choose to call themselves lesbians because it is easier, and because they do not want to acknowledge their bisexuality, to themselves or to others. The possibility of stigma from bisexuality leads some women to call themselves lesbian.

For others, it is a matter of context. Many women in the study reported that sex with men "doesn't count" as salient to identity for a number of reasons. Context is important here. For some women, identifying with the queer community outweighs the gender of sex partners when self-labeling. According to one woman, "I can sleep with men all I want, but I don't connect. I don't want relationships with them." Some women experiment sexually with men just for the experience. For others, it was the goal that mattered. They want different things from sex with men and women. Several women said that with men, sex was casual. It was just sex, there was no emotional connection, and they did not want a relationship with a man. Therefore, the actions were not salient to the identity label. According to one woman, who said she called herself lesbian for simplicity's sake, "I've never dated guys in a long-term thing, just more casual. I want the free meal and the free fuck kind of thing." Since she did not consider men seriously as far as dating, it was easier to just call herself a lesbian. This was similar to Cara, a twenty-one-year-old single white woman who called herself a lesbian, who said she prefers to have relationships with women, and enjoyed sexual activity with both women and men.

INTERVIEWER: Can you tell me a little bit about why you consider yourself to be a lesbian?

CARA: Because I prefer to have relationships with women, and because I enjoy sexual activity with women.

INTERVIEWER: You also said that at this time you would be willing to have sex with both men and women?

CARA: I'm embarrassed to say that because of coming out. I feel like I went all through this struggle, and I thought the attraction to men, that I questioned that because it's never quite as good, and I don't want to be in a long-term sexual relationship with them. So it's like men have their place. I don't consider myself bisexual because I don't consider men and women equally, what I want from them.

INTERVIEWER: Okay, so what do you want from men?

CARA: Gratification.

INTERVIEWER: And from women?

CARA: Friendship, love, sex, the whole shebang.

Cara said she did not consider herself bisexual because she did not consider men and women on the same level. From men, she was seeking physical pleasure; from women she wanted friendship, love, and sex. She was embarrassed to say she would have sex with men because of being out as a lesbian. Becca, a thirty-one-year-old white woman who identified as lesbian and lived with a long-term female partner, was also open to the idea of having sex with a man under the right circumstances. She described her feelings toward sex with men:

INTERVIEWER: Since you've been out, have you slept with men?

BECCA: No, but I certainly wouldn't rule it out. I personally believe that sexual orientation is on a continuum, and while earlier in my life, because of denial, I practiced having sex with men as part of my sexual life, there might be another time. I can see myself being open-minded enough that if I saw another person who happened to be a male, I wouldn't say, "Well, I'm a lesbian, I can't do this." If

I was in love with a person and I wanted to have sex with them, I would. Right now my primary partner's a female, and that's not an issue at this moment.

For Becca, as for others, identifying as lesbian did not mean she would never have sex with men.

Another context in which a lesbian might have sex with men is during the coming-out process. Becca referred to this as denial. We are all socialized to be heterosexual, and having sex with men is often just part of a larger socialization. Guilt about being a lesbian may lead a woman to have sex with a man during coming out. Ebony, a twenty-three-year-old African-American, single woman who identified as lesbian, described it this way:

EBONY: I went through—one of my friends called it the denial-slut stage.

INTERVIEWER: The denial-slut stage?

EBONY: Yeah, because it was, when I started realizing that I like women, I was afraid I was a lesbian. So in order to prove I wasn't, I started sleeping around with guys a lot. It was bad, really bad.

INTERVIEWER: Was this when you were in high school?

EBONY: In high school. When I'd first start falling for a girl, I'd run out and find a guy.

This is often transitory, and as the woman solidifies her self-identity she often stops having sex with men. Coming out is a process, and women handle it differently. Michelle, a twenty-four-year-old single white woman, described her choice of identity label when coming out in this way:

Lots of people call themselves bisexual when they come out, because it is too scary. I felt less comfortable [calling myself bisexual] because I felt I wanted to identify with a queer community and bisexual is not socially acceptable in a lot of parts of queer communities. I wanted to be unequivocally identified with a lesbian community.

Another woman was just coming out as a lesbian at the time of the study. She was under twenty-one and, although she had sex with men and had not yet had sex with a woman, she identified as lesbian. As identity and actions are fluid, women sometimes go from identifying and acting as a lesbian to a shift in identity and engaging in sex with men. Two women in a focus group had this conversation about being married to men and how that plays into their feelings and actions toward their same-sex attractions:

INTERVIEWER: Okay, since you brought up being married to a boy, why don't we talk about what is your sexual orientation? Do you have a label for it? Do you consider yourself to be in one category? How do you define that?

LOTTIE: Well, I define myself as either bisexual or queer, depending on the day.

INTERVIEWER: Does that change over time?

LOTTIE: It has very much changed over time. For the past three or four years I would say I've defined myself as bisexual, but before that I defined myself as a dyke.

JESSIE: Now that you're married, is that like a commitment-commitment?

LOTTIE: Yes.

JESSIE: So you don't plan on jumping back over the fence?

LOTTIE: That's a fair question.

JESSIE: You met him, he was everything you ever wanted in a person, right?

LOTTIE: Right. Which isn't to say I haven't been with women.

JESSIE: Since you've been married?

LOTTIE: Yeah.

JESSIE: Okay, okay [laughter]. That will be fine.

KAILA: Here, I'll help you out, because I'm married to a boy, too. And it's very tempting sometimes to go out with my friends, and you go, "She's soooo cute and she's flirting with me." It's really hard. It's really hard sometimes.

Lottie and Kaila had both engaged in relationships and sex with women in the past, and Lottie continued to engage in same-sex sexual activity after her marriage to a man. Kaila, too, was still attracted to women, but had not had sex with women since her marriage. Their identities and actions changed over time, and both acknowledged that they may continue to change over time.

Other reasons why lesbians have sex with men include pressure from family to be heterosexual and the desire to have children. More contexts in which lesbians have sex with men include sex work, exchanging sex for food or rent, and cheating. One couple said they cheated on each other with men in order to get pregnant, and also when they prostituted for food or money. They still identified as lesbian and said the sex with men did not count because it was goal-oriented and not part of their identity. One woman conjectured that, "If you're gay but you're sleeping with men, it is probably because you want the experience. Either they just want to experiment, or they're having a hard time, or they're being pressured by their family or whatever." Identity is related to risk. Maureen, a focus-group participant, described how she conceives of identity and risk:

> If your partner has done IV drugs or whatever. There's like the check marks in the boxes. When it comes down to it, anything can expose you. There's all these questions of, like, potency and frequency, and all this other stuff that is supposed to factor in. But I think that overall when you're talking about in the greater lesbian community, the point is that the public discussion outside of health and activism of lesbians and sex health has not really come out at all except in the last couple of years, really. I mean, regardless of activism that's been going on for a while in a group like Safe Sex Sluts and things like that, when it comes right down to it, in general, it's still not actively promoted that women need to be protecting themselves against other women—whatever that might entail. This whole idea of separating identity and behavior is the fact that I could be lesbian-identified and tomorrow I could go out and have sex with a man and that could put me at risk and it could put a female partner at risk. It is just not something that we want to think about. It's not that it's

not there, it's just that we don't want to deal with it, I think, in a lot of cases.

Maureen was especially knowledgeable about lesbian sexual risk because she is a sexual-health advocate. She is aware that, often, identity does not fully describe behavior. This incongruence that is often found between identity and actions can have several consequences. A label does not necessarily equal internalized identity, nor does it always correspond with actions. Refusing to acknowledge one's behavioral tendencies can put one at risk for HIV or STIs, especially if those actions are ignored or marginalized as irrelevant to one's identity.

Many lesbians seem to want to stick to a rigid definition of what it means to be a lesbian, and they often assume that everyone else defines labels in the same way. One woman responded to a query on her thoughts about lesbians who have sex with men with this: "Whatever. It's their choice. But I don't think they're lesbians; I think they're bisexuals." If a woman thinks that identity labels and actions are the same, and does not question this further, she may be putting herself at risk. If a woman defines lesbian as a woman who has sex exclusively with women, and her partner calls herself lesbian, she may not question further, because she assumes that they are both defining in the same way. People often lie and omit relevant information in the context of sexual relationships. One woman, acknowledging this, also acknowledged that protecting oneself from STIs and HIV is one's own responsibility: "I think if they are having sex with men, they should tell their sex partner. But I don't think that's going to happen. I mean, maybe, but I don't think so. So it's your own risk. Sex is your own risk, really." Also, many STIs do not manifest in detectable symptoms, especially in women, and these infections can be passed from one woman to another without either woman being aware of the transmission.

Some women view others whose actions do not directly match their sexual identity as misleading or dishonest. They seem to feel that a person should call herself what she is or, in the case of sexuality, what she does. This can decrease confusion and allow women to make more informed and conscious choices about their sex partners and sex acts. Although some women who identified as lesbian did not mind when women were bisexual, they viewed it as positive if that bi-sexuality was disclosed. Other women who identify as lesbian will not view anyone who has sex with men as a potential partner. Debbie, a twenty-six-year-old white woman who identifies as a lesbian, described her feelings this way:

INTERVIEWER: Okay, how do you feel about lesbians who have sex with men?

DEBBIE: My feelings have changed recently, and part of me still feels like I really don't care who someone else is sleeping with, but I wouldn't want to be in a relationship with someone who had recently been sleeping with a man. But I don't know. I really am having a hard time with this one. My partner is transgendered, and so we have lots of issues in our relationship about women sleeping with men. It's a really big deal, big issue. And I never really thought about it, I actually slept with other men, not just that guy I dated, not many, three other men. And they were like a one-time-each kind of thing. And I was really having a hard time, and lots of things were happening, and it's been a long time, though. And then like the other lesbians going through the same thing, I have no problem with that, because I can understand it. And I always thought before that it really didn't have anything to do with their sexuality. I mean, who you're having sex with doesn't always have to do with your sexuality; there's a lot of other things that influence you. But at the same time, I think that it probably has more to do with stability than anything else.

INTERVIEWER: Being afraid that they would go back to sleeping with men?

DEBBIE: I wouldn't want to date someone that was bisexual, because I don't want to be left for a man. And that's just an ego thing. But if they're really gay, I think if you're gay but you're sleeping with men, it's probably because, well, it could be just because you want the experience, but I think that happens when people are younger and not older. Either they just want to experiment, and they don't need to be in a relationship anyway, or they're having a hard time, or they're being pressured by their family or whatever, then they're not very stable, either. I have no problems being friends with them, I just don't want to sleep with them.

Debbie was aware of the reasons some lesbians have sex with men, and did not stigmatize them for it in terms of friendship, but she did not want to have sex with a woman who is having sex with a man. Debbie acknowledged that choice of sex partner is not always about sexual identity.

SEXUAL ACTION IN BIOGRAPHICAL CONTEXT

So what is it lesbians actually do in bed? This may be the most common question asked by nonlesbians about lesbians. The larger cultural definition of sex tends to be very phallocentric. Sex that does not involve a penis, specifically penile-vaginal penetration, is often not even defined as sex. People therefore have a difficult time grasping that lesbian sex (in the absence of a penis) is indeed sex. In this heterosexist context, even sexual activity between men and women that is not intercourse is often labeled as foreplay rather than as sex. This rigid definition of sex potentially puts many people at risk. For example, consider this question and answer printed in a nationally syndicated sex-advice column, "Savage Love" (Savage, 2001):

Dear Dan:

You say in your recent column that the only way to truly avoid STIs is to not have sex [Aug. 8]. Well, a friend of mine contracted genital herpes (at the time, she was a virgin) from a guy who went down on her while he had a herpes breakout in his mouth.

Catherine

Everybody, all together: Oral sex is sex. . . . Your "virgin" friend was just as sexually active as any crusty ol' dyke, and all sexually active people put themselves at some risk of contracting STIs. . . . It's the price of admission. Giving or receiving, there are a number of STIs that can be contracted through oral sex. . . . While the risk of contracting HIV while performing oral sex is very low . . . the relative rarity of oral HIV transmission comes as cold comfort to people who were infected that way.

This advice column illustrates how, even among heterosexual people, sex is not easy to define. Misconceptions and misinformation can contribute to risky actions.

Table 3.2 indicates the sexual activities in which women in this sample said they have participated. I asked respondents when was the last time, if ever, they had participated in certain sexual activities, either with men or with women. The list is by no means exhaustive; I did not ask about many common lesbian sexual activities that did not pose a risk for HIV or STI transmission. See books such as *The Lesbian Sex Book* (Caster, 1993) for a description of a whole range of lesbian sexual activities. Only the activities that potentially pose a risk for HIV or STI transmission are shown in Table 3.2.

The majority of the sample (79 percent) had had vaginal sex with a man at some point in their lives. This is similar to other research findings of 70 percent (Diamant et al., 1999). For most, however (58 percent), it had been more than a year since they had done so. Only 12 percent had had vaginal sex with a man in the three months prior to the interview, and another 9 percent in the four to twelve months prior to that. Contrarily, 69 percent had had vaginal sex with a woman (defined as penetration by fingers, hands, or objects such as a dildo) in

TABLE 3.2. Sexual Activities of Respondents

Activity	Never	>1 Year	4-12 Months	Past 3 Months	No Answer
	Percentage (N)				
Last vaginal sex with man	21 (33)	58 (94)	9 (15)	12 (20)	0 (0)
Last vaginal sex with woman	2 (3)	10 (16)	19 (31)	68 (111)	1 (1)
Last oral sex with man	29 (47)	54 (87)	6 (11)	10 (16)	1 (1)
Last oral sex with woman	4 (6)	14 (24)	20 (32)	60 (97)	2 (3)
Last woman oral sex with you	4 (7)	15 (25)	21 (34)	59 (95)	1 (1)

the three months prior to the interview, and another 19 percent in the four to twelve months prior to that. In only 10 percent of the sample had it been over a year, and only 2 percent had never participated in vaginal sex with a woman.

Nearly 30 percent of the women had never performed oral sex on a man. This is slightly less than Diamant and colleagues' (1999) finding of 38 percent. For another 54 percent, it had been more than a year. Only 10 percent had engaged in oral sex with a man in the three months prior to the interview, and another 6 percent in the four to twelve months prior. For many women, this sexual activity with men had happened prior to their coming out as a lesbian or during a behaviorally bisexual period during their coming out.

Most of the women (80 percent) had performed oral sex on a woman in the year prior to the interview (60 percent in the prior three months, another 20 percent in the four to twelve months prior). Only 4 percent had never performed oral sex on a woman. The breakdown was almost identical for the last time a woman had performed oral sex on the respondent. I failed to ask about men performing oral sex on respondents, so I cannot compare use of protection between male and female partners.

Because several studies mentioned it as a phenomenon, and because it is a high-risk sexual activity, I also asked about penetrative anal sex with men. Most study participants (75 percent) had never participated in penetrative anal sex with a man. However, nearly 25 percent had, and for 5 percent it had been within the prior year. Another study showed 17 percent as ever having anal sex with a man (Diamant et al., 1999). For other activities that could potentially pose a risk, I simply asked whether the respondent had ever engaged in each activity. Table 3.3 shows the results of this questioning.

Oral sex during menstruation can pose an increased risk compared with other times because of the added factor of blood, which can be ingested or which can come into contact with abrasions in the mouth. (Some people advise not to brush one's teeth before having oral sex because vaginal or menstrual fluids can potentially enter the bloodstream through small abrasions.) About half of the women had performed oral-genital sex on a menstruating partner. This was twice as many as the 23 percent found in another study (Myer, 1997). Almost 60 percent had had digital penetrative sex with a menstruating wom-

TABLE 3.3. Past Behaviors

Have You Ever:	Yes (%)	(N)
Had oral sex on a menstruating woman?	49	(78)
Had digital sex with a menstruating woman?	60	(93)
Fisted another woman?	30	(47)
Been fisted?	23	(37)
Inserted sex toys into your vagina?	75	(121)
Rubbed genitals with female partner?	97	(155)
Had oral-anal contact?	46	(73)

an, which could potentially put blood in contact with any abrasions on hands or around fingernails.

Fisting is a sex act whereby one partner inserts a whole hand into the vaginal cavity of another. As this stretches the vaginal walls, there is a potential for tearing. Nearly 30 percent of respondents had fisted another woman, and 23 percent had been fisted. This was much more than the 8 percent giving and 8 percent receiving in another study (Myer, 1997).

Three quarters of the respondents had inserted sex toys into their vagina, and many of these women shared their sex toys with a female partner, thereby potentially transferring vaginal secretions. Nearly half had had oral-anal contact (anal rimming), a route of transmission for hepatitis. Tribadism, or rubbing genitals, is an extremely common behavior (97 percent) in woman-to-woman sex among the sample. This is often a direct, sustained rubbing contact of mucous membranes and skin, which is a direct route of transmission for several sexually transmitted infections. These numbers were also higher than the 64 percent found in another study (Myer, 1997).

Respondents also answered questions about sex work, or sex exchange. Five percent (N = 8) had given drugs or money for sex, and 13 percent (N = 21) had given sex for drugs, money, food, or a place to stay in the year prior to the interview. Richters and colleagues (1998) found that 9 percent of the 585 women recruited at a gay festival had exchanged sex in the year prior to the study. With regard to sex toys, 70 percent of this sample had used a dildo, and 29 percent had used vibrators. Seventy-one percent of those who had used sex toys reported sharing them with their partner.

Lesbian women engage in a variety of sexual actions. This is somewhat contrary to the popular perception that lesbians do not engage in activities which may pose a risk. However, women in this sample engaged in an array of actions which could potentially transmit HIV or sexually transmitted infections. These include sex with men, drug use, oral sex, sex during menstruation, sharing sex toys, and rubbing genitals. Any of these activities could potentially put one in contact with another's vaginal fluids or blood.

Chapter 4

Constructions of Risk and Protection

I describe Helen, a thirty-three-year-old African-American woman, to illustrate someone with multiple risk factors.

Helen had a history of risky actions, showed a lack of control in her sex life, and frequently failed to utilize protection. Helen had been raped. She had been homeless and vulnerable. She was a drug user and a sex worker. She met her last female partner in jail (her cellmate). Helen had been pregnant more than four times, had three teenaged children, and did not have custody of them. At the time of the study, Helen was in drug treatment and resided in a halfway house. Helen had a high school diploma and worked full time but made less than $10,000 a year. She was single and defined herself as from an upper-class background. Both she and past partners have cheated on one another.

Helen said she is very likely to ask about drug use, STIs, and AIDS with potential partners. She claimed to be in very good health, and although she did not have a regular doctor, she did have a regular place to go for health care: a women's clinic. She also received care at a family planning clinic and at a community clinic. She had no health insurance. Helen said she always disclosed her sexual identity (bisexual) to health care providers. She had received care for trichomoniasis in the year prior to the interview.

Helen had sex with both men and women, and identified as bisexual. She was out to her family but not to all of her friends. She first had sex with another female when she was twelve years old. Her first sexual intercourse with a male took place at age sixteen. She had sex with both men and women in the six months prior to the interview. Although Helen claimed to always use condoms when having vaginal sex with men, she did not use a condom the last time she had vaginal sex with a man. She said, however, that she planned to always use condoms with men. Helen never used gloves for digital sex with a woman and never used condoms on sex toys. She said she always used condoms when giving oral sex to a man but never used dental dams or other barriers when giving or receiving oral sex with a woman, although she said she planned to start doing so.

Helen said she did not perform oral sex on menstruating women. Helen had never had anal sex with a man. She engaged in tribadism and sometimes had sex while high on drugs. In the year prior to the interview, Helen frequently exchanged sex with men for money, drugs, or goods. She has had multiple partners and has had sex with someone she knew injected drugs. The times when Helen did not use protection, she said it was because she forgot. She has had occasions where her vagina was dry to the point of bleeding during sex. Helen said her friends talk about protection much more than they actually use it.

Helen had used crack, heroin, and marijuana, and was a casual alcohol user. She attended Alcoholics Anonymous or Narcotics Anonymous meetings almost daily. She had been in drug treatment three times, both long-term inpatient care and outpatient care. Helen had been tested for HIV ten times in the five years prior to the interview. She was tested at a clinic, at a health department testing site, in jail, and in drug treatment. She was HIV negative and thought her chances of getting AIDS were "none." She said that she and her relatives and friends did not talk about AIDS. She displayed some knowledge about HIV transmission, although she did think you can tell if someone is HIV positive by looking at them and that smoking crack does not put people at risk for HIV transmission.

Helen had been attacked, beaten, and raped. Although Helen had been in a variety of risky situations and had engaged in an array of potentially risky behaviors, she continued to assert that her risk of acquiring HIV was none. She did not view herself as susceptible. If Helen, with multiple risk factors, did not consider herself to be susceptible, would other women with fewer risks consider themselves as such? What factors cause lesbians to view themselves as susceptible? In this chapter, I discuss respondents' constructions of susceptibility, followed by their constructions of risk and protective factors. Finally, I discuss barriers to reducing risk. Many of the women in the study exhibited at least some of these risk actions, yet most (70 percent) considered their HIV risk to be low, and another 16 percent considered their risk to be none. Table 4.1 shows the results of this question.

I asked respondents about HIV and STI statuses. Here, I will briefly provide descriptive frequencies regarding HIV and STIs. One hundred forty-two women (88 percent) had been tested for HIV. Of those, seven women (5 percent) reported that they were HIV positive. In addition, 23 percent of respondents (N = 36) had had a diagnosis of a sexually transmitted infection sometime in their lives. Six of the HIV-positive women were among the 23 percent that had been diagnosed with an STI. Fourteen of the women (37 percent) who had been diagnosed with an STI reported exchanging sex in the year prior to

TABLE 4.1. Chances of Getting AIDS

What Do You Think Your Chances Are of Getting AIDS?	Percentage	N
None	16	26
Low	70	112
Medium	8	14
High	4	7
No answer	2	3

the interview. Among those who had been diagnosed with a sexually transmitted infection, 50 percent (N = 18) identified as lesbian. The sexually transmitted infections that were reported included genital herpes (twelve cases), trichomoniasis (eight cases), genital warts or HPV (five cases), gonorrhea (four cases), chlamydia (four cases), syphilis (two cases), and crabs (one case). One limitation of these data is that the survey did not allow respondents to report having been diagnosed with more than one infection, so these numbers may not include all cases of each type of infection.

STI rates for the general population are difficult to estimate. Many STIs manifest with few or no symptoms, and individuals might self-treat an infection and not visit a doctor for diagnosis. Nevertheless, the CDC does provide prevalence data for some STIs. According to the Centers for Disease Control and Prevention (1999), in 1999 chlamydia rates for women were 404.5 per 100,000. For gonorrhea, the rate for women was 136 cases per 100,000. Syphilis cases were 14.3 per 100,000 women. HPV rates were unavailable, as the CDC reported that they were too difficult to diagnose and track.

PERCEPTIONS OF SUSCEPTIBILITY TO STIs AND HIV

How do lesbians construct their picture of personal susceptibility? Three groups developed among this sample: women who feel invulnerable, who are either unaware of the risks or refuse to admit that it can happen to them; women who are aware of risks and take steps to protect themselves; and women who seem to be aware of the risks but who do not choose to protect themselves. For a few, the possibility of contracting a sexually transmitted infection seemed inevitable, so they did not use protection. Several of these women were in long-term relationships with a woman who had an STI or who was HIV positive.

Invulnerable

Kahala (1999) found that lesbians see themselves, to an extent, as immune to HIV contraction. She found that this construction of invulnerability was based on sexual behavior, the association of risk with bisexual women and with men, and on community values and stereotypes. Similarly, many women in my study felt that they were not susceptible to STIs or HIV simply by virtue of being a lesbian. Several women stated that "you can't get anything from a woman." This reflects a larger cultural myth that lesbians are not vulnerable to sexually transmitted infections. One woman said it was a known "perk" of being a lesbian. There seems to be a feeling of invulnerability based on myths such as an "amazon sisterhood" or "cosmic protection" for lesbians. Sally, a thirty-seven-year-old, African-American, divorced woman who considered herself a lesbian, described it in this exchange:

INTERVIEWER: You also mentioned that you haven't used any kind of protection with a woman and that was primarily because you have been in long-term monogamous relationships. What kind of behavior do lesbians engage in that might be considered risky?

SALLY: When I look at my friends, both casual and close, I think that there is an issue with number of partners. Especially since I think that more lesbians than not have had some sexual contact with men. Younger ones are less likely. It's just amazing how early women are figuring out that they are lesbians whereas my generation went through a period where there was a lot of thinking about it and going back and forth with it. But I still did see a lot of bisexuality and a lot of discussion of bisexuality that leads me to believe that we aren't as open about it, perhaps because we aren't accepting about it. In that sense, the number of partners and the probability that more are sleeping with men, that combination is risky.

INTERVIEWER: What about women who are just sleeping with women, are they risky amongst themselves?

SALLY: You asked a few questions about my friends and whether or not they talk about protecting themselves. I think they actually do, but there really isn't very much discussion about it. I think I'm pretty guilty of this too, and I don't know how I would behave in a new relationship, but my suspicion is that I would not think very much about protection under the circumstances. That may be because after about a year of knowing them I would engage in intimate behavior with them. But I think we still assume that the risks are low and that there is something special about women and the relationships that we have that offers some kind of cosmic protection. I really do believe there is this need to feel that we are so different and so special and that we are blessed in some way with some powers to protect ourselves, and I think that is a part of it. Even the cases where there is a connection there are still doubts about those, so it's hard to convince people that this is important and that they have to do it.

Sally described a desire to be part of a special group. One feature of this special group is their safety from HIV and STIs, which are common in other groups. Although she was aware that this sense of "cosmic protection" was a construction, Sally still felt some sense of invulnerability.

Many women in this study reported that they had never heard of a woman getting an STI from another woman, as well as that they did not know much about safer sex with women and neither did their friends. Another notion that leads women to feeling invulnerable is believing that if a woman looks healthy, she is healthy. According to one woman, who has unprotected sex with men and with women and who also smokes crack, "People never ask [about STIs]. Because I run, I think they assume that I am healthy and that I don't do drugs. They assume if you look healthy you don't do anything unhealthy. Wrong." Also, if a woman calls herself a lesbian, there is often an assumption that she is, by virtue of that label, infection-free. Many lesbians feel that bisexual women are STI "carriers" and so avoid having sex with women who self-label as bisexual to avoid risk. For other women, it was the definition of risk itself that may put them at risk.

One woman, who described herself as a lesbian, had unprotected sex with both men and women and did not tell her women partners about her sex with men. She felt that the sex with men was random and since she would never see them again, she did not need to inform her other partners about that activity. Since there is often little exchange of fluids with women (and no risk of pregnancy) they saw no need for protection. Heather, a forty-four-year-old white woman who considered herself a lesbian, described her thoughts this way:

> When I think of protection I think of a long time ago when you worried about gonorrhea and syphilis and then you worried about being pregnant, so in a lesbian relationship I'm not worried about pregnancy and then with STIs I'm trusting fate, which is kind of not that smart. I don't want to sit there and fuss with all this plastic when I'm having sex.

Another woman said she didn't use protection with women because, "There's nothing that squirts up inside of me." She reported using condoms with men, but not always, and she had been pregnant several times and smoked crack. Neither woman felt vulnerable to HIV or STIs, and neither took precautions. However, both engaged in potentially risky activities.

Several women simply said they were not at risk because they, and their communities, were not promiscuous and were selective about their partners. Other women saw only male partners as being risky for STIs, and if they were not themselves having sex with men, then they were not worrying about it. These women did not view sex with women as being risky or themselves as being susceptible. Some women evaluate the need for safety based on the specific sex act, rather than on the partner. Jill, a twenty-six-year-old single white woman, said the following:

> Well, I use condoms with men when I have sex, when I have vaginal intercourse or anal intercourse. If I was having sex with my boyfriend and he was going down on me or fingering me, I wouldn't use protection then, either. I guess it's not necessarily the person I'm having sex with, it's the act I'm doing. I guess

maybe it's easier to get HIV when semen is shooting up into you than it is when your girlfriend's fingering you and she's got a cut on her finger.

For others, it was never even a concern. One woman said, "I never thought about asking if [partners] had ever been tested for anything. That never even occurred to me. It had only occurred to me to find out about the relationship part, not the sex part." Another woman said, "With women, I really don't think that AIDS is a big enough threat to warrant having to use protection. I don't ever hear of any lesbians getting STIs from each other." Becca, who is aware of risk factors, described the invulnerability issue in this way:

> The image is that lesbian means I've never touched a man, and never will. And a sort of hypothetical Amazon sisterhood, where we're all perfectly well behaved, none of us use drugs, none of us share blood, and it's just totally safe. None of us are into penetration. We all just hang out. We're sexual somehow, but there are no risk factors.

Although this may not be a consciously held belief, it does appear prevalent. This group of women have a culturally constructed sense of invulnerability based on the group to which they belong. They feel that, as lesbians, they are invulnerable to contracting HIV or STIs.

Aware and Protective

In contrast to the invulnerable group, a second group of women was very well educated about sexual risk factors for lesbians and regularly took protective actions. Two were safer-sex educators in the lesbian community, and others had either had firsthand experience or had known lesbians with STIs. This group of women evaluated potential partners based on a number of factors, then made an informed choice as to whether they felt they needed to use protection. Some women define a partner as low risk if she does not have sex with men, is not an IDU, and has been selective with her partners. The number of partners a woman has had plays an important role with this group, as increased numbers of partners suggest a greater risk of having come into contact with an STI. One woman said, "I think there is an

issue with number of partners. Especially since I think that more lesbians than not have had some sexual contact with men. But we aren't
as open about it because we are not accepting about it." If a woman
from this group does not know whom her partner has been sexually
active with, she feels susceptible. Stella, a twenty-eight-year-old
African-American woman who has a steady female partner, described how she evaluates risk:

> I would think that a woman who goes down on another woman
> is at greater risk because there's more virus, viral load, what-
> ever. And the vaginal secretions versus saliva. It's my under-
> standing that saliva is so low that it's not really a concern. So
> anyway, but I do know that there's always the risk of cuts in your
> mouth, or from flossing, or your toothbrush has slipped. Reus-
> ing toys that may have blood or vaginal secretions on them.
> Again, I am saying this only for people whose history you don't
> know, or you do know that they have a history that puts them at
> risk.

Stella had different standards for protection based on her knowledge
of a partner's sexual history. Participants mentioned other risk factors, including having multiple partners, using drugs, and identifying
as bisexual.

Some women were aware that often identity and actions do not
match. Annette, a twenty-seven-year-old white woman who identifies as queer, shared her thoughts on this.

> There are people who identify as lesbian but at the same time
> have male partners. There are lesbians who live full-time with
> female partners but have sex with men either for money or what-
> ever, but they still identify as lesbian. So I think that kind of
> skews everything off, and women have fluids so they can pass
> [infections] on to each other.

One interesting subgroup in the lesbian community is the S&M
community. Several women in this study were involved in this subgroup, and they described participants as among the safest people
with whom to have sex. According to one such woman, "The women
that are into the S&M community are like the safest, into very safe

sex, because generally they have multiple partners and they're just really the safest, nicest people." Overall, the women in this group of aware and protective actors showed a deep understanding of the potential risks involved and actively took preventive measures.

Aware in the Abstract

In addition to the invulnerable group and the aware and protective group is a third group who are abstractly aware of the risk, but who do not feel personally susceptible. Some lesbian women steadfastly stick to the position that although some lesbians do contract STIs, it is not a personal issue. They simply do not accept that they are at risk, keeping their eyes closed to the information they report having. In this group there is a general refusal of personal susceptibility, even when aware of the risk factors. Sometimes it simply does not occur to them to even ask their potential partners about STIs. They may assume that if a potential partner has an infection then she will disclose that before having sex. However, the women who did have STIs had different ways of handling disclosure. Among the women who reported already having an STI, attitudes toward disclosure differed. Some women told every potential partner of their infection and insisted on using protection during sex. Some said that facing the stigma and ignorance of others led them to not disclose their infection to partners. Others simply seemed unaware that transmission to a woman was possible. For example, when I asked one woman who had genital warts if she ever worried about giving these warts to a woman, she replied, "No, I haven't. Do you think I should?" Genital warts can be passed by skin contact.

Another woman (who had genital herpes) said she overheard a woman saying she chose to have sex with women because "you can't get anything [infections] from them." "And I'm standing there with herpes, you know, next to my lover who doesn't have it yet, and one of the biggest things we've had to face in our relationship is her not getting it and here is this woman saying you can't get shit from each other." She was very frustrated at the lack of knowledge that she perceived among lesbians and the hidden nature of lesbian STIs. The minimization of risk can be frustrating to women who are aware and protective. Most of the women who were in the aware in the abstract group did not see themselves as personally susceptible because of the group they belong to, who they perceive their partners to be, or what they perceive to be risky actions.

With regard to personal susceptibility, the women in this study fell into three groups: those who felt that they were invulnerable, those who were aware and protective, and those who were aware in the abstract yet refused to acknowledge personal risk. The women who felt themselves to be invulnerable may not have been consciously thinking of themselves as such. Often, the feeling of invulnerability was subconscious. Some respondents simply never thought about it. For many, it was an assumption they made based on group affiliation. Lesbians are generally thought to be at low risk for contracting HIV and STIs, and that belief has become part of the lesbian cultural group's stock of knowledge. Often, the status of lesbian is constructed as protective in and of itself. Those who were aware of potential risks and took protective actions initiated these actions in a context in which they might not have been welcome, as they were acting against the larger group's beliefs. The third group was aware of risks but denied that they were personally susceptible. This refusal may be a way of handling potential discomfort about discussing STIs or utilizing protective techniques.

One's attitude regarding susceptibility will affect one's perceptions of risk and protection. A woman who feels personally susceptible will be more likely to recognize potential risk and utilize protective actions. A woman who feels invulnerable may, in contrast, engage in risky behaviors because she refuses to acknowledge that she, personally, may be at risk as a consequence of her actions. Those who are aware of the risks but feel that they are not valid concerns for them may tend to engage in potentially risky behaviors in the context of that refusal.

Chapter 5

Risk and Protection

I asked study participants to describe what they thought were risky actions and what measures they find sufficient for protecting themselves. Responses varied. Having sex outside of a relationship can be a risk factor. Regarding relationship fidelity, 65 percent of respondents had felt that at some point, a partner had cheated on them. Fifty-six percent had cheated on a partner. Thirty-two percent had ever been pregnant, but 63 percent want a child at some point. Of those, 17 percent planned to become pregnant through sex, 16 percent through an at-home insemination (potentially risky, as the semen is not tested for HIV), 15 percent through a clinic insemination, and 53 percent said they did not know how they were going to get pregnant. Depending on how a woman decides to get pregnant, she may or may not be placing herself at risk. Sperm banks and clinics are probably not as risky as at-home insemination or as having sex with a man to get pregnant.

Communication is paramount in reducing risk and increasing protective actions. It is important to know a partner's history so as to be aware of risk factors and to be informed to take appropriate protective measures. The women in this sample reported a high level of communication with partners, and often this communication was considered to be sufficient protection. I asked how likely they were to ask partners about drug use, STIs, AIDS, and past sex partners. Although many women were comfortable bringing up these issues with partners, others were not. One woman said, "I guess I am not really comfortable just flat out asking, you know, 'So, what's your sexual history? Have you been tested for AIDS?'" Table 5.1 shows the response to "How likely are you to ask a potential partner about the following?"

TABLE 5.1. Asking About Risk Factors

How Likely Are You to Ask a Potential Partner About the Following:	Very Likely	Somewhat Likely	Unlikely
	Percentage (N)		
Drug use	69 (112)	24 (38)	7 (12)
STIs	63 (103)	20 (32)	17 (27)
AIDS	71 (115)	13 (21)	16 (26)
Past sex partners	63 (102)	27 (44)	10 (16)

Although most women reported asking potential partners about these factors, many did not. Not gathering relevant information about a sex partner's history of risk factors can potentially put one at risk.

A number of factors other than actual sexual actions may put a lesbian woman at risk. These include community beliefs, definitions of risk, and social constructions of what constitutes safety. Community beliefs may influence risk-taking in that they are an inherited body of knowledge which is often taken for granted as being accurate when, in fact, parts are often based on misconceptions or stereotypes. Definitions of risk are more individual. I asked respondents to tell me what actions they thought could put them at risk for infection. Similarly, I asked respondents to describe what protective measures they found sufficient in their own lives.

Community-held beliefs that influence risk-taking include ideas about bisexual women, about the community itself, and about the nature of safer sex. There seemed to be a general belief among the women in this sample that bisexual women were a bridge carrying STIs from the straight community to the lesbian community, a view which is supported in the literature (Marrazzo, 2000b). They were sometimes referred to as disease carriers, often in ways that villainized those women who disclose that they are bisexual. They are often also seen as being dangerous romantically, as they may alternate between male and female partners. Tavis, a thirty-seven-year-old African-American lesbian who has never had an STI, explained:

INTERVIEWER: If you identify as exclusively lesbian, would it bother you if your partner said she was bisexual?

TAVIS: It wouldn't bother me, but I would rather not date a woman that's bisexual. To be perfectly honest, I think we're all bisexual, I mean, everyone. It's just that we get to a point where we make a decision and we stick to that. . . . And I think that chances of STDs are higher when you're involved with men, personally.

This conception of bisexual women can deter those who are bisexual from disclosing their sexuality to female partners. One woman said, "I had just as many problems coming out as bisexual to my queer friends as I had coming out the first time." These women often feel pressured or stigmatized for their identity and disclosure of that identity.

Lesbians comprise only a small segment of society, with limited numbers of potential partners. Like most people, they tend to select partners from their social networks (Richters et al., 1998), and respondents reported what they referred to as an "incestuous community." One woman described the network as comprised of "two degrees of separation," in that everyone eventually dates or has sex with many other women in the circle, and two people who are dating are also likely to have past partners in common. She said this during a focus-group discussion:

> And the two degrees of separation is so true. There's that girl I slept with, and then she slept with my ex-girlfriend. It's amazing, the chain; it's such an incestuous relationship. You figure everybody has slept with everybody through one or two people.

Also, women reported having multiple partners and believing that others do, as well. This is viewed as a potential risk, as it is likely to increase the possibility of transmission. If one person in the network has an infection, others in the network are likely to eventually become infected as well. Conversely, if a circle is somewhat closed, and no members have infections, the network might serve as protection.

Another prevailing belief is that safer sex among women is too bothersome. Women in another study (Kral et al., 1997) said that lesbian safer-sex techniques were awkward, not readily available, and expensive. In this study, the methods were described as "stupid," "confusing," "too much trouble," "less enjoyable," and as a potentially offensive topic. Ebony described confusion like this:

> It is not as cut-and-dried with women as it is with men. I mean, like, with men, use a condom—boom—that's it. With women, you can use a glove, you can use Saran Wrap, you can use a dental dam, you can cut a condom open, you can do all this stuff. With guys, there's the immediate thing with pregnancy there and that whole body-fluid thing that's there. That's a very real thing that you have to deal with, so of course you're going to use something to be contained, it's just something you have to work around.

When comparing safer sex with men to safer sex with women, taking action with male partners seems more clear-cut and necessary.

One woman said she and her partner experimented with dental dams for fun and it was "not so fun. It was so silly, and I couldn't imagine having sex with someone and having to do all that. I don't know how to make it feel good." Another woman viewed sex as an "all-or-nothing" deal, reflecting a belief that barrier protection got in the way of a complete sexual experience.

> Okay, I'm having sex with a girl, right? And, you know, we're going down on each other, and she's fingering me, and whatever. Why wash the dildo? Because, I mean, I don't use dental dams, and I don't use finger condoms and all that, then what's the point? So, if I am going to get something, I am going to get something.

Some women said they were offended if a partner asked them to use protection, because it made them feel somehow unclean, as if they were suspected of having an infection. For example, I asked Anne, a thirty-five-year-old single white woman, how she thought she would feel if someone pulled out a glove during sex.

> Oh, I'd be completely offended. A glove! Oh, my God! I would think we probably shouldn't be having sex. I would be so turned off. I would be like, "We need to just stop if that's the way you feel." A glove, God, like you're going into surgery or something.

Another woman said that although she does not have an STI, when she suggests using condoms on sex toys, her partners assume she does. Others said they were wary of asking partners to use protection because they did not want to offend them. However, one woman described being impressed when a partner raised the issue:

> I was so psyched because it's happened several different times and every time I think that is so cool that [they] have enough self-esteem and respect to just lay it out there and to put aside insecurities and assumptions and just be like, "This is what it's about. This is what I need. What do you think? Here it is."

For others, it was a matter of comfort and sensuality: "I just analyzed where I'm willing to go, what feels good and tastes good and what doesn't affect it. I really enjoy oral sex and the feeling and the taste without barriers. And the same thing with digital." For her, and others, safer sex meant decreased pleasure.

When respondents described how they conceptualized risk, the answers fell into two categories: sex-related risks and non-sex-related risks. Sex-related risks included oral sex with sores in the mouth, penetrative vaginal sex with open cuts on fingers, unprotected vaginal or anal sex with men, unprotected sex with a man for the purpose of pregnancy, and oral sex on a menstruating woman. One woman said she would not perform oral sex on a menstruating woman but that her partners do perform oral sex on her while she is menstruating. She says this is "their choice." All of these actions are commonly recognized as risk factors among lesbian health advocates. Very few women mentioned the "scissors" position, where rubbing genitals together can provide transmission opportunities, although one woman reported transmitting an STI to a female partner in that way. Another woman brought up anal rimming, saying "there is always fecal matter and bacteria issues. It's just not hygienic." She uses split condoms for barrier protection.

Most women did not bring up non-sex-related risks, but the ones that were mentioned are important. People who are sex partners and who also use drugs will often use drugs together. Sharing crack pipes or needles was mentioned as risky. Sharing crack pipes can result in blood being passed from one person's mouth to another's when burning and bleeding occur. One woman said clean needles are hard to get in the United States, and it was hard to clean them. As she just did not want to clean them, she shared with partners in the past. Kral and colleagues (1997) found that 53 percent of women who have sex with other women and also inject drugs reported sharing needles. Other risky actions that were mentioned as taking place in relationships were at-home piercing, sharing razors, and sharing toothbrushes. Betty, a forty-five-year-old white woman who had trichomoniasis and hepatitis C, raised the issue of sharing razors, and although she did not think she could transmit hepatitis sexually, she was not sure whether a partner who used a razor after her could be infected.

> Someone could come over and decide to get a little romantic, and maybe you've been out all day rollerblading. Let's take a shower, and somebody decides to maybe buff up and shave around their leg or something, and the other girl comes into the shower and shaves. If one is positive, whether it is HIV or hepatitis C or hepatitis B or a number of different things that are bloodborne, using the same razor, she could get it that way. Maybe she decides to clip her fingernails. That's the way it could get transmitted. Sharing a toothbrush can get [it] transmitted. Those are things that I could see happening. When people decide to become sexual, things like that go out the window.

Similarly, she noted how sharing toothbrushes could potentially pass blood from small cuts in one person's mouth to the other person. Betty was the only respondent who raised the issue of razors and toothbrushes. Respondents showed awareness of what constituted risky actions. For the most part, they knew which specific sexual actions could potentially be risky. Since they were aware of many risks, I asked them whether and how they protected themselves from risk. The next section describes protective lines of action.

PROTECTIVE LINES OF ACTION

In addition to asking what are considered risky actions, I also asked respondents to describe what they thought were sufficient protective measures with regard to STI and HIV transmission. For some women, the answer was that they do nothing. For many others, trust seemed to play a big role. Asking one's partner about her sexual history was often viewed as sufficient protection. One woman said, "I'm into total history, and I'm not ashamed to talk about it." Another woman, who had sex with both men and women, said she does not use condoms with men, "But I haven't ever fooled around with a man whose sexual history I didn't know and feel confident about." She felt that if she knew her partner's sexual history, she would not be at risk. Others replied that they have only long-term partners and are serially monogamous. The belief was that if they did not have multiple partners then they were not at risk. Using safer-sex strategies when having sex with someone they know is bisexual is one protective strategy. However, some women who identified as bisexual were reluctant to disclose that to partners because they did not want to acknowledge their own bisexuality. This lack of knowledge can limit their partners' protective lines of action. Some bisexual women said they took sexual risks because they did not want to acknowledge their own sexuality and also to avoid the guilt and stigma that is associated with disclosing that they are bisexual.

Very few women used protection all the time, although some did. Others used it when they thought they were with a high-risk partner or in a high-risk situation. One woman contracted herpes from a partner who did not disclose her status. "I was told after having sex with somebody that they had herpes. I was pissed off. I mean, it's no problem if they told me, and I needed to be educated about it." She did not find out about her partner's herpes infection until her partner had an outbreak. She felt that if she had known about her partner's infection, she could have initiated a different protective line of action. Many women did not think that protection was necessary. One focus-group exchange articulated feelings about taking protective actions.

EMMA: I don't think it's important. And after being somewhat, at least, educated I still don't think so. And that may be the wrong answer statistically etcetera, etcetera, but it just, and I'm one of those serial monogamous, I date one person, and usually feel like I know them, and I usually do. And I'm not shy about asking questions, and you know, especially in a relationship for awhile, and I know this person's sexual history, you know, feel totally safe in all ways.

But in general I feel like it's just not as important, the health risks are low for HIV transmission between women, and other STDs, although other STDs I think are more easily transmitted. And I feel like I have the knowledge to go, "Oh, you've got genital herpes, it's important." Then I would protect myself. But as a general thing, no.

POLLY: I agree. I'm pretty monogamous. I'm very monogamous when I'm in relationships, and I would never have random, you know, just go home with someone, and I know it's not about just going home. It's more just like she said, ask questions. I always ask questions. I know the person I'm sleeping with. But I don't think I could do it unless I knew the person. Chances are, if I knew the person had something, I probably would not. I mean, unless I was in love. I don't know, it's a complicated situation.

IMANI: Are you saying that if you asked and they said they had a disease, you would not date them?

POLLY: If I was in love with the person. If it was a dating situation, then I probably would not want to have a physical relationship. If I were to fall in love with that person, that would be different.

IMANI: What if you fell in love with them, then found out they had it?

POLLY: That would be difficult. I would hate to be exposed to something like that. Once you have herpes and a lot of those things, you just can't cure them. I wouldn't want them to have any of that.

EMMA: Even though I had, I have had a one night stand with someone I knew, but didn't know their sexual history, and even in that case it would have crossed my mind had it been a man, for sure. But because it was a woman, and then she was someone I knew as a friend, you know, it didn't cross my mind. And I never really looked.

FANNIE: I think it depends what you do. I think in certain instances it is important. Like all those questions that answered, being a medical student, I would think it would be really important if you were being physical when one of the two partners was menstruating. I think that would be really important to have protection then. But otherwise, I don't. Yeah, I would be really careful about men, like no condom, no sex.

These women were not ambivalent about the risk and protective actions they were taking. They see risk in the abstract, but they do not appear too worried about their own personal risk. Polly said she would not have a physical relationship with a woman she knew had an STI, and she was still hesitant when someone asked her what she would do if she fell in love with a person who was infected. There is a feeling that avoiding sex with an infected person would eliminate the risk. That would be true if all STIs were detectable and if all sex partners were honest in their disclosure. That is not always the case.

Several women who had an STI or HIV discussed the measures they deemed sufficient for preventing transmission to their female partners. One woman who had herpes said she always disclosed her condition to partners prior to engaging in sexual activity and that her partners rarely elected to use safer-sex strategies. Another woman, who was HIV positive, said the same thing. She disclosed and left it up to the partner to decide whether to utilize protective measures. In addition to unprotected sex with women, she also had unprotected sex with multiple male partners. Most of her female partners opted not to use safer sex. One respondent mistakenly believed that she had HIV and during that time had unprotected sex with her partner. "I went home and had completely unprotected sex with my partner, and I put her completely at risk." She also did not disclose what she believed to be her status to her partner. She felt that since she had already been sleeping with her for months, her partner had probably already contracted the infection from her.

Allison, a white lesbian woman with herpes, described the stigma that accompanied telling potential partners. When she told someone about her condition, a rumor subsequently started in her community that she was HIV positive, a rumor she said persisted for eight years and very much affected her life. After that, she chose not to disclose her herpes. To try to avoid transmitting to a partner, she would not have sex while she was having an outbreak. At the time of the interview, she was in a relationship and I asked her, if she were to date, how she would handle disclosure of her herpes infection to potential dates. She answered this and told how she discovered the rumor about herself.

ALLISON: We're talking about today, right? Right now, today, I don't want to be with anybody else. And if it comes to the point where I have to accept that fact that we're not together, it's hard to say. Because it makes you not want to tell people, and I do know that I will date longer without the physical contact, before, you know, but I can't say what will happen. I mean, I've experienced someone who, once I told them [I had herpes], spread a rumor that I had AIDS.

INTERVIEWER: How did that affect your life, the rumor?

ALLISON: Well, at first I didn't know for sure. I knew she had said something because all of a sudden everyone in the community was like, standoffish, looking at me strange, you know. You can tell when people are talking about you. But it hurt, and I didn't find out until, actually a woman that I was in a very abusive relationship with told me that's what it was. She said, "People are talking about you." I was like, "What do you mean?" And she told me, "They're saying you have AIDS." And that's why we took the test, when I went to [the hospital], I was like, "I don't have a problem taking the test."

INTERVIEWER: Was she afraid that you would hide it from her?

ALLISON: She was afraid, period, because the sexual part of our relationship was never her doing anything to me. And maybe that's all part of her anger, too, I don't know. But why would you get in a relationship even though you hear all the talk, I don't know.

Allison's partner had heard rumors that she was HIV positive, and therefore she did not perform potentially risky sexual actions on Allison. She also requested that Allison be tested for HIV, which Allison was glad to do, to dispel the rumor that she was HIV positive. One HIV-positive woman prefers to have sex only with other HIV-positive women: "I like being with someone HIV positive because I don't have to go to all the trouble of meeting someone I care about and having to go into, 'Well, hey, I'm HIV positive,' and they take off and run. I'm more comfortable with someone who's positive."

Protective lines of action include not only communicating and abstaining from potentially risky sex but also actively taking protective measures such as using actual barriers (usually latex) during sex. I asked women questions about protective actions they took in general. Table 5.2 shows the results of this questioning.

TABLE 5.2. Protective Actions

In General:	Never (N)	Rarely (N)	Sometimes (N)	Always (N)	Total (N)
			Percentage (N)		
When you have vaginal sex with a man, how often do you use a condom?	28 (40)	11 (15)	23 (33)	38 (54)	142
When you have vaginal sex with a woman, how often do you use gloves or a condom?	52 (81)	19 (30)	18 (29)	11 (17)	157
When you have oral sex on a man, how often do you use a condom?	75 (104)	9 (13)	9 (12)	7 (10)	139
When you have oral sex on a woman, how often do you use a dental dam or other barrier?	80 (129)	11 (17)	7 (11)	2 (4)	161
When a woman has oral sex on you, how often do you use a dental dam or barrier?	82 (131)	11 (18)	6 (9)	1 (2)	160
When you have oral sex on a menstruating woman, how often do you use a dental dam or other barrier?	93 (145)	3 (5)	2 (3)	2 (3)	156
When you have anal sex with a man, how often do you use a condom?	43 (21)	6 (3)	1 (9)	33 (16)	49

Note: Row totals do not add up to 162 because not all of the respondents engaged in each behavior. Percentages reflect row totals.

Very few women in this sample said they always use protective barriers during sex. The number was highest (38 percent of those who have had sex with men) for those who used condoms when having vaginal sex with men, which is perceived as the highest risk as far as sexual activity. This is also related to condom use for pregnancy prevention. The next highest use of protection (33 percent) occurred among women having anal sex with men. Other studies found that lesbians who had sex with men rarely used protection for vaginal sex: only 18 percent (Diamant et al., 1999), 40 percent (Marrazzo, 2000a), and 17 percent (Norman et al., 1996).

The most striking results are from the "never" category. More than one-quarter (28 percent) of the women who have had vaginal sex with men report never using condoms. Almost half of those who have had anal sex with men never used condoms, and three-quarters of the women who have performed oral sex on men did not use condoms. Most (93 percent) women who performed oral sex on a menstruating woman never used a dental dam or other barrier, similar to the 80 percent who never use barrier protection during nonmenstrual oral sex. The only woman-to-woman sexual activity for which a large number (48 percent) of women used protection was using gloves or a condom at least rarely during vaginal sex with a woman. When asked about the last time they had vaginal sex, only 54 percent of respondents reported using a condom the last time they had vaginal sex with a man, and 20 percent reported using gloves or a condom the last time they had vaginal sex with a woman. One woman described her feelings this way: "I don't particularly care for all these precautions, measures. Although I understand that they are a necessity to some extent, I don't like them." Other factors besides the use of condoms, dental dams, or other barrier protection are important elements in evaluating risk. The context in which sex occurs and the history of one's partner are important. Table 5.3 shows the results for other past-year risky actions.

TABLE 5.3. Past-Year Risky Actions

In the Past Year, Have You:	Yes (%)	N
Had sex while high on drugs or alcohol?	85	135
Had sex while your partner was high on drugs or alcohol?	85	135
Had sex with a man who may have had sex with another man?	15	23
Given money, goods, or drugs for sex?	5	8
Given sex for money, goods, or drugs?	13	21
Had sex with a partner who had injected drugs?	12	20
Had sex with someone you knew had purchased sex?	10	16

Alcohol and drug use can be an important factor in risky actions, and a correlation has been shown in the literature. Alcohol and marijuana consumption among lesbians is associated with increased sex risks (Kahala, 1999), increased anonymous sex, and sex outside of one's relationship (Perry, 1994, 1995). Most women in this sample (85 percent) had sex while high on drugs or alcohol in the year prior to the interview, and the same percentage had sex with a partner who was high on drugs or alcohol. Drugs or alcohol can reduce one's inhibitions, make one less selective with partners (for example, sex with strangers), and can lead to less use of protection. Some people may use alcohol to avoid awareness of sexual risk (Perry, 1994). Alcohol can also reduce one's self-control and control over the situation. One woman described being forced to have (unprotected) sex with a man while under the influence of alcohol. She was out with a male friend, and she was drunk. He threatened to rape her if she did not perform oral sex on him. "And if I hadn't been drunk, I would have known, okay, there's other ways to get out of this, but I just freaked and thought, *Okay, if I give him a blow job, he'll leave.*" Alcohol diminished her ability to make clear protective decisions.

Injection-drug use is a means of transmission of HIV and other infections, which can then also be transmitted sexually. Twelve percent of the sample had sex in the prior year with someone they knew had injected drugs. Einhorn and Polgar (1994) found that 10 percent of self-identified lesbians and 15 percent of bisexual women had had sex with an injection-drug user. Fethers and colleagues (2000) found that 21 percent had done so. Fifteen percent of this sample had sex with a man who may have had sex with another man. Because male homosexual sex is a primary means of HIV transmission in the United States, this action may put these women at risk.

Sex exchange is another risky context. Women who exchange sex may have less control over protective actions. Having sex with someone who has purchased sex may also put one at risk. Ten percent of the sample had sex in the prior year with someone they knew had purchased sex. Thirteen percent had traded sex for money, goods, or drugs in the prior year, and 5 percent had given money, goods, or drugs for sex. Fethers and colleagues (2000) found that 22 percent of their sample of WSWs had ever exchanged sex. In addition, 20 percent (N = 33) of this study's respondents had, in their lifetimes, had sex with someone they knew had an STI, and 4 percent (N = 7) had at least one sexual partner they knew was HIV positive. Kral and colleagues (1997) proposed that sex work and lesbian identity interact in a subgroup of lesbians who have sex with men only in the context of sex work.

The women in this sample listed many behaviors that could potentially lead to risk. These included sex acts and nonsex actions related to relationships. These also included choice of sex partner, number of sex partners, sex-partner networks, drug and alcohol use, and sex exchange.

Most (88 percent) of the respondents had been tested for HIV at least once, indicating that lesbian women are concerned about HIV. This is higher than the 48 percent of respondents tested in another study (Perry, 1994). HIV testing is viewed as a protective action. Because most of the women said they were at low or no risk for HIV, I asked why they were getting tested. Table 5.4 shows the results of these questions.

Slightly more than half (56 percent) were tested because they thought they had put themselves at risk. For some, the risk was unprotected sex with someone they did not know well. For others, it was a work-related incident, such as one health care worker who had been scratched in the eye by a patient. One woman knew she was at risk for HIV but was too scared to get tested and potentially get a positive result. She felt at risk because of having had sex with an IDU, having had multiple partners, and having had sex with a woman who was married to a gay man.

Where do lesbian women go for HIV testing? Many of the women in our sample were tested more than once, sometimes at different places. Table 5.5 shows HIV testing sites. When respondents who

TABLE 5.4. Reasons for HIV Testing

Were You Ever Tested Because:	Yes (%)	N
You thought you were at risk?	56	75
It was suggested by a health care professional?	22	30
You had an HIV-positive partner?	2	3
You felt sick and didn't know why?	5	7
Your partner wanted you to?	13	18
You were pregnant?	6	8
It was part of a treatment program?	7	10

TABLE 5.5. HIV Testing Sites

Were You Ever Tested At the Following:	Yes (%)	N
Clinic or hospital	49	66
Emergency room	7	9
Gynecologist	10	13
Private doctor	31	42
Health department	36	49
Jail	3	4
Drug treatment	9	12

had never been tested for HIV were asked why they had not been tested, they reported that they knew they were not infected, they never thought about it, they didn't want to know, or they did not know where to go.

The women in this sample showed a high level of knowledge about risks and protective actions. They generally viewed protective actions as necessary in certain circumstances, yet they generally did not practice protective behaviors and did not always avoid risky actions. Whether individuals view themselves as susceptible, at risk, and in need of protective actions is affected by their perceptions of risk and protection, by their sexual identity, and by barriers to utilization of protection. In the next section, I describe such barriers.

TYPICAL BARRIERS TO PROTECTION

Barbara was twenty five years old, white, single, and had some college. She worked full time and made between $25,000 to $35,000 per year. Her job included health insurance, and she had a regular doctor. Barbara had no children and had never been pregnant. She wanted children eventually, but was not sure what method she would use to get pregnant. She always came out to her health care providers. Barbara was treated for genital herpes in the year prior to the study.

Barbara chose the label of bisexual for the purposes of our questioning but said, "I don't like the term *bisexual.* I don't like to be labeled. I just consider myself the kind of person who enjoys the company of different people." She first had sex with a man at the age of eighteen. She knew she was interested in having a relationship with a woman but did not know how to go about coming out. Her first sexual relationship with a woman occurred about a year before the interview. Barbara was not sexually active at the time of the interview. She had, in the prior year, disclosed her sexuality to family, friends, and her doctor.

Barbara said she always used condoms when she had sex with men but had never used any sort of protection when she had sex with women, which included oral sex, digital sex, and genital rubbing. She used sex toys but did not use condoms with them. She had, at least once in the prior year, a tear or cut in her vagina that bled from sexual activity. She said she did not use protection with women because she felt it was too much of a bother.

Barbara had used powder cocaine and marijuana. She had taken one HIV test (which was negative), at her private doctor's office, because her female partner suggested that she be tested. She felt she was at low risk for HIV contraction. The first time Barbara had sex with a woman, they discussed HIV and STIs. She told her partner that she had herpes prior to sexual contact, and they did not use any barrier protection. When asked if she had ever had any sex that she would consider risky, Barbara tellingly answered, "No. Well, in some ways I've had it several times. I got herpes." Barbara knew that the male partner from whom she contracted herpes had the disease, but she chose not to use condoms when he did not have a visible outbreak. Barbara felt responsible for the transmission, because she was aware of the risk and chose not to use protection.

At the time of the interview, Barbara had just started dating a woman. They had not yet had sex, and Barbara had not yet told her partner about her herpes. She said disclosing her STI was a difficult thing to do:

> Yeah. Not that I don't want to tell her. It just has to do with my life. I have a lot going on and relationship and sex is quite low on my priority list and having to go into it means having to have emotional talks and because I don't need or want the relationship thing it's almost a relief to me to know I don't have to go into it with anyone right now. But it's hard. Even though I've accepted it, it's still hard to look someone in the face. Because you don't always know someone and how they look at you. I don't really want to go there if I don't have to, but over maybe the next few weeks or months I could change my mind depending on how far along this thing goes.

Barbara was afraid of a negative reaction and relieved that she did not yet have to tell the woman she was dating that she had herpes. Although Barbara had contracted herpes, she still tended to think that she had not engaged in risky actions. This was true for many women in the survey, who felt that they were not at risk yet engaged in potentially risky behaviors. Several themes emerged from this study regarding barriers to utilizing protective measures. These included institutional barriers, interpersonal barriers, circumstantial barriers, and labeling barriers. Institutional barriers include a lack of sex education in high school and even in college regarding lesbian sex, which can lead to skewed knowledge on lesbian HIV and STI risks. I asked respondents where they got their information on lesbian safer sex. The list included gay festivals, jail, AIDS organizations, friends, partners, a feminist health center, and a rented educational video. Lotta, a focus-group participant, put it this way:

LOTTA: You don't get taught it. It's basically talking with friends. Actually, there was a video I saw about lesbian safe sex. It came out a few years ago; I don't remember the name of it, but it was an educational video about that.

INTERVIEWER: Where did you see it?

LOTTA: I worked in a movie store, and that was probably the only reason I realized it was there. They stuck it back in the porn section [laughter]. It in a way was [porn], but it should have been more in the educational section.

The list did not include private doctors or school- or college-based sex education programs. Other institutional barriers include being closeted to health care providers with regard to one's sexuality. This can potentially be a barrier because of internalized homophobia or fear, real or perceived homophobia on the part of the health care providers, or because some health care providers would not think to ask questions about same-sex sexual behavior.

Interpersonal barriers include communication issues. Many women prefer to avoid the topic of STIs because they are scared, embarrassed, or shy about bringing it up. Some women lie about their status because they either do not want to acknowledge it or they do not want to face potential stigma. One woman said that by the time she and her most recent partner had progressed to riskier sexual actions, they were breaking up, so they did not ever talk about it. Circumstantial barriers come into play in the context of alcohol or drug use, jail, rape, and sex work. One respondent who had spent time in jail said that when exchanging sex there for food and other goods, she felt she had little control in the situation and could not utilize protective measures. Identity and action were discussed earlier; the divergence that often occurs between the two can be a barrier to utilizing protection. Again, the notion that lesbians are somehow "cosmically" protected comes into play, as does "intuitive trust" when some women claim that safer sex is unnecessary when they feel comfortable or connected with a partner.

For many women, lack of access to reliable health care and health information can be a barrier to reducing risk. Among this sample, 40 percent had no regular health care facility and 51 percent did not have a regular doctor. Fifty-four percent had had health insurance for the entire year prior to the interview, and 27 percent had not had insurance for any of the prior year. Almost all had at some point had a routine medical exam (94 percent), a pelvic exam (94 percent), and a pap smear (94 percent).

Disclosing one's sexual identity to one's health care professional can be an important protective mechanism. Most respondents (66 percent) at least usually disclosed this information, although some did not. One respondent described a recent visit to her doctor for a yeast infection:

> Whatever the hell it was [the cause of the infection] she's like, so geared toward men about where I got it and why it was irritated or whatever. It's bullshit for me to be lying to her. I was lying to her the whole time.

See Table 5.6 for more data from respondents regarding their disclosure to health care providers.

Even if a woman does come out to her health care provider she may not get appropriate information, and in some cases the assumptions the doctor makes about her sexual behavior, along with the resulting lack of knowledge on the woman's part, may put her at risk. One woman said her doctor told her she did not need to get pap smears if she was really having sex only with women. Marrazzo (2000a) strongly recommends that the pap regimen for women who have sex with women should not differ from that of heterosexual women. Paps screen for HPV, and 19 percent of the women in their sample who had never had sex with a man were found to have HPV. In my study, another woman's doctor, even after being informed that she was a lesbian, continued to focus on her reproductive health and the only re-

TABLE 5.6. Disclosure to Health Care Providers

Do You Come Out to Your Health Care Providers:	Percentage	N
Never?	9	14
Rarely?	4	7
Sometimes?	20	33
Usually?	25	40
Always?	40	64
No answer	2	4

sponse to her disclosure was, "I have a bunch of gay friends." One respondent, who always discloses her sexual identity to health care professionals, finds that it limits the care she receives. "I've been to a couple of different doctors, and once they realize I am a lesbian, discussions about any STIs or pregnancy . . . they simply find that nonapplicable and discussions don't take place." Her experience was similar to that of the respondent who asked her doctor at the women's health center how to prevent passing genital warts and herpes to her partner. Her doctor said she did not know and gave her the number to a lesbian hotline, which she never called. Diamant and colleagues (1999) found that health care providers may not solicit a comprehensive sexual history from lesbians because of assumptions about their activities based on their label.

Many women do not take protective actions during sex. Table 5.7 shows the reasons why women in this sample did not use protection.

Research shows the importance of knowing or trusting one's partner, intuition, and self-esteem in choosing not to utilize safer sex (Kahala, 1999). Although many women in my sample indicated that they often did not know why they failed to use protection or that they did not think it was necessary for lesbians (I failed to put that as a choice) almost half (47 percent) said it was because they trusted their partner or were in a long-term relationship.

Most women had an open attitude toward protection (see Table 5.8) and said they would use protection if a partner wanted them to.

TABLE 5.7. Reasons Cited for Not Using Condoms or Dental Dams

When You Did Not Use Protection, Was it Because:	Yes (%)	N
You trusted your partner or were in a long-term relationship?	47	77
It was too much of a bother?	26	43
Other?	6	9
You were not planning on having sex?	8	12
You forgot?	6	9
You were embarrassed to ask?	1	2
You asked, and your partner refused?	1	1
You were afraid you would not get paid?	1	2
You were afraid your partner would refuse or abuse you?	1	2
No answer	3	5

TABLE 5.8. Attitude Toward Using Protection

Attitude	Disagree	Neutral	Agree	No answer
		Percentage (N)		
Would object if a partner suggested using protection	66 (107)	16 (26)	16 (25)	2 (4)
Has difficulty saying no to partner	59 (95)	15 (25)	25 (41)	1 (1)
Would avoid using protection if at all possible	57 (93)	19 (31)	22 (35)	2 (3)

Although most women showed a willingness to engage in protective actions, many did not actually do so. A lack of knowledge can potentially place one at risk, so I also asked respondents to answer some basic HIV/AIDS knowledge questions. Most showed a solid factual foundation. See Table 5.9 for those results. The only question that a significant percent of the sample missed regarded the risk from smoking crack. Since it is not a direct risk, many women did not see the

TABLE 5.9. HIV/AIDS Knowledge

Statement	Correct Answer	Percent Correct
You can tell from looking at a person if they have the virus.	False	91.4
A negative test for HIV does not necessarily mean you do not have HIV infection.	True	95.1
It is possible for a baby to get HIV from breast-feeding if the mother is HIV positive.	True	65.4
Using a condom can reduce your chances of becoming infected with HIV.	True	98.8
HIV, the virus that causes AIDS, is present in semen, blood, and vaginal fluids.	True	98.1
Smoking crack does not place you at risk for HIV infection.	False	54.9
A woman cannot get HIV from sexual contact with another woman.	False	90.7

connection. Hot pipes can result in cracked or bleeding lips, and sharing pipes can pass blood from one person to another. Stephanie, a twenty-nine-year-old African-American woman who identifies as gay, said she had a medium risk for acquiring HIV. When asked why she thought it was medium, she replied, "Because when I was out there messing around I had a likely chance because of me using a pipe. I wasn't using protection on the pipe." There also may be a link between crack use and sex exchange. In addition, drug use is described in the literature as being associated with unsafe or risky behaviors. I asked respondents about their drug use history (see Table 5.10). Most women (83 percent) had used marijuana at some point in their lives. Almost half (42 percent) had used powder cocaine, and nearly one-third had used speed (33 percent) or crack cocaine (32 percent). Only 11 percent had ever used heroin.

Only 10 percent had ever injected drugs, and only one respondent had injected in the year prior to the interview. This is similar to the 12 percent who used injection drugs in the past six months in another study (Richters et al., 1998). Many of the women in my study who had used drugs reported a change in their selectivity of partners (see Table 5.11), with heroin having the biggest impact. Fifty percent of

TABLE 5.10. Drug Use

Have You Ever Used:	Yes (%)	N
Crack cocaine?	32	51
Powder cocaine?	42	68
Heroin?	11	18
Speed?	33	53
Marijuana?	83	134

TABLE 5.11. Drug Impact on Partner Selectivity

How Does _____ Impact Your Selection of Partners?	Less Selective	More Selective	No Change
	Percentage (N)		
Heroin	50 (5)	20 (2)	30 (3)
Cocaine	32 (18)	13 (7)	55 (31)
Speed	27 (10)	8 (3)	65 (24)

those users reported that it made them less selective with their partners. Some women did not have sex while they used the reported drugs.

Having sex while using drugs can lower inhibitions and allow people to act in ways they would not ordinarily act if they were not using drugs. One woman said drugs "make you do things you never thought you would do, and I didn't care because I was trying to get high." Another described the effect of alcohol use on her sex life in this way:

> There are times you are just drinking until you are really blitzed and you end up falling in with somebody and you're not really aware of sex or even if you consider using barriers, you are so drunk and sloppy that it isn't effective.

It is clear that alcohol or drug use can decrease protective behaviors.

Barriers to protection included institutional barriers, interpersonal barriers, circumstantial barriers, and labeling barriers. Health care practitioners who are ill- or underinformed can mislead patients into thinking they do not need to worry about sexual risks from sex with women. Interpersonal barriers, such as a lack of communication, can also lead to risky situations. Having sex in the context of using drugs may inhibit one's control and the actions one takes. Given the constructions of susceptibility and the perceptions of risk and protection, what factors will lead lesbian women to change their actions to reduce risk and utilize protective behaviors?

ANTICIPATED LINES OF SEXUAL ACTION

Given what these women know about risk and protection, what are their future plans for utilizing self-protective actions in terms of safer sex? Table 5.12 shows plans for safer sex. Most respondents were still not planning to use barrier protection when having sex with other women.

According to the health belief model, when one is aware of risk and protective factors and is aware of being susceptible, and the benefits of reducing risk appear to be greater than the cost, an individual will take protective actions. This does not necessarily seem to be the case here. The benefits to utilizing safer-sex procedures sound good, but the costs appear prohibitive. In addition, although the women in this study generally showed a high level of understanding of HIV and STI risks, they often did not think they were personally susceptible. I asked women what circumstances have changed or would change their stance on this. Several women said that getting a sexually transmitted infection or HIV changed their stance. Others did not change until they transmitted an infection to a partner. For example, one woman transmitted herpes to a partner and says she now plans to be monogamous in order to not spread her infection to anyone else. Another woman contracted genital warts and now plans to use plastic wrap as a barrier when receiving oral sex. Plastic wrap is often suggested by safe-sex educators as a cheaper and more readily available alternative to dental dams. Several women said that until they participated in this study, they were unaware of risks and, as a consequence of their participation, would now start taking more protective actions. One woman described how her sexual stance changed dramatically

TABLE 5.12. Plans for Protective Action

Do You Plan to Use:	No	Maybe, Unlikely	Maybe, Likely	Yes	Don't Plan Sex with a Man
	Percentage (N)				
A condom every time you have vaginal sex with a man?	8 (12)	2 (4)	2 (4)	25 (40)	63 (102)
A condom every time you perform oral sex on a man?	8 (13)	8 (12)	2 (4)	9 (15)	73 (118)

Do You Plan to Use:	No	Maybe, Unlikely	Maybe, Likely	Yes	Don't Plan Sex with a Woman
	Percentage (N)				
Condoms or gloves every time you have vaginal sex with a woman?	34 (55)	36 (59)	11 (18)	14 (23)	5 (9)
Dental dams every time you have oral sex with a woman?	40 (64)	39 (63)	11 (18)	7 (11)	3 (6)

after she found out she had hepatitis C: "I'm very careful. Strictly no sex. When I found out I had it, it just completely surprised me. I haven't come out of that, so I'm like this walking contaminated thing." Her response also speaks to the stigma and guilt associated with infections. Stigma and guilt also can lead to taking protective lines of action.

Other women mentioned more general factors as having changed their stance. For example, increased awareness from the AIDS epidemic, personal friends dying of AIDS, and hearing about lesbians and STIs from friends have led some women to be more cautious. One focus-group participant described how working in the area of HIV had affected her perceptions:

> I have known so many people who have or have had HIV who have died. Countless, countless numbers of people. That's just it. I don't ever play unsafe. There's no such thing as unsafe sex in my world. It's one thing if you're monogamous. If you decide to be, like, fluid bonded with someone, that's a commitment you want to make, and you have both been tested, and tested again.

Some women changed their stance when a partner asked them to use safer-sex techniques or to get screened for HIV or STIs before commencing a sexual relationship. Others said if they knew a partner had an STI they would still have sex but would use barrier protection. A few people mentioned one-night stands as a temporary shift of stance. One woman said, "It would take her [sex partner] saying that she'd either slept with a lot of women, or sex with a lot of people she didn't know. If a woman told me she had an STD, I would probably not sleep with her." One woman said she has stopped having sex that involves direct contact altogether.

Considerations that led or may lead to change among the women in this sample varied. Contracting HIV or a sexually transmitted infection was one such factor. Although some women with STIs do not disclose their status to their sex partners or do not utilize protective actions to reduce the risk of transmitting to their partner, many women with STIs were strongly affected by acquiring the infection and were steadfast in their determination not to infect others. Some women had sex with a partner who they knew had an infection and still did not feel personally vulnerable and did not use protection. Others said they plan to change their actions and use protection if they have a partner with an STI. Still others would refuse to have sex with a person they knew to be infected. Other women planned to change their actions when they became personally involved with HIV-positive people and were alarmed by the severity of the disease when they saw it firsthand.

Constructions of susceptibility included invulnerable, aware and protective, and aware in the abstract. These constructions are informed by one's sexual identity, one's sexual actions, and one's perceptions of risk and protection. Although the women in this study generally understood what actions could lead to transmission, they still frequently did not utilize protective actions, many viewing communication and partner screening as sufficient protective actions.

TALKING ABOUT RISK:
FOCUS-GROUP CONVERSATIONS

Several of the themes discussed in this chapter are revealed in the conversations lesbian women have among themselves, found in the comments of women in the focus groups. Individuals in each of these groups showed an awareness of potential risk and protective actions. Two groups included a lesbian safer-sex advocate. The first group also included a virologist. Another group's discussion focused on dental dams and where to get them, including jail. These women's unique positions gave each of them an awareness and knowledge that others in the lesbian community may not share.

INTERVIEWER: When you had sex for the first time were you thinking about the fact that there might be certain health risks? What, if anything, would you consider unsafe lesbian sex today?

JESSIE: I guess it all is. I mean, unless you know the history of whomever. Seriously. Because any of the fluids that are exchanged can carry HIV, or whatever.

TESS: Yeah, I think that's how my attitudes have changed. I came out in '76, so, you know, I was a young dyke running around, sleeping around with any woman who would sleep with me. There weren't really any issues in my mind. STDs weren't a factor. HIV wasn't around or known about then. Whereas as the HIV epidemic got going, I became very aware of health risks, and that started, not necessarily altering my sexual practices, but I think not being quite as promiscuous as I had been previously. And, you know, not going to the bar and picking up a woman, and going home for a one-night stand, which had been sort of part of my practice at one stage. And now I'm in a committed relationship . . . damn! [Laughter.] When I started dating this woman, even prior to that, it was always, "I really like you, and the relationship has moved to a point. However, I'm not going to bed with you until we've each had an HIV test." And then also discussing previous histories, you know, "Do you have genital herpes? Have you had gonorrhea?" From that, tests come back negative, and then pursuing a sexual relationship. Working in—I had done a lot of AIDS activism in the early stages of the epidemic. Also, I am a virologist, so my area of work, I deal with blood products all day, every day, so I'm exposed to HIV on a regular basis. I was aware, and I wasn't prepared to take chances on either side. But I don't think that's common among the lesbian community.

Tess's stance on her own vulnerability changed over time, and that change was accompanied by changes in her actions. Early on, she did not think the risk of infection was significant and she took no protective actions. They were simply irrelevant. The HIV epidemic and her involvement as an activist altered her awareness of vulnerability. This awareness led to changes in protective actions that Tess considered unusual for lesbians in general. Later, her career as a virologist placed her in a position where she had to be up to date on HIV knowledge. She feels less vulnerable because of her extensive knowledge. I then asked others in the group about their experience with HIV testing, which led to an impromptu miniworkshop on safer sex, led by Maureen, the activist.

INTERVIEWER: Has anybody else had that experience of getting an HIV test with a partner? With a female partner?

LOTTIE: I had a female partner who wouldn't have sex with me until we did [have an HIV test]. And it [sex] was extremely latex laden, even though we both came out negative.

JESSIE: Even after taking the test?

LOTTIE: Yeah.

INTERVIEWER: How did that make you feel?

JESSIE: Because I have done that, but I didn't know if that would be safe! [Laughter.]

INTERVIEWER: Has anybody ever taken a mint condom and cut it and used that as a dental dam?

MAUREEN: Well, I do a safe-sex workshop with some other people, so, in that respect, yes I have. But otherwise I haven't.

INTERVIEWER: Can you tell us about that?

MAUREEN: There's a few of us. One a public-health person who has been doing activism for about five years [inaudible], and there's myself, and two seniors in college, and my . . . ex used to be in the group with us as well. But we don't do that anymore [laughter]. And, basically, we go to colleges, conferences, groups that ask us to come (queer groups), and model all types of behaviors. It's very much based on behavior rather than identity. We play with toys, and show people how to use lube, and do this sort of neat starter at the beginning where everybody puts a glove on and pours some lube on and rubs hands with the people next to them. It's a way to say, "Okay, it can feel kind of good." And everybody's sort of going, "Eww. . . ." It gets a little freaky for people sometimes when I pull a big dildo out of my pants, and things like that . . . [laughter].

JESSIE: Could you do that now? [Laughter.]

MAUREEN: Of course, it is not with us right now! [Laughter.] But that's the kind of stuff we do. It's sex positive, a lot of times youth focused, and we try to stay away from medicalized terminology because we find it too alienating. We just encourage people to be interactive, to volunteer to model stuff, whatever it happens to be.

JESSIE: How would you use this [indicating the condom]?

TESS: The only problem is they always come with spermicide.

INTERVIEWER: It's flavored for oral sex.

KAILA: See, but everybody talks about it, but does anybody use it in real life?

MAUREEN: [Demonstrating] Normally, you would have a little reservoir, but basically you just cut the tip off and unroll it, and cut it down the side and open it up.

JESSIE: Oh, okay.

MAUREEN: It's cheaper.

JESSIE: Then what do you do?

MAUREEN: You can try to hold it yourself, but that gets a little sketchy. You can have your partner hold it, or you can get a cute little harness.

JESSIE: On the genitalia or in your mouth?

MAUREEN: Over the genitalia. The harnesses are kind of cute. You can get a black leather one—those are nice. They'll just fasten it and strap around the girl's legs. Or, you can use Saran Wrap, which is kind of nice because you can just wrap it around and it sticks by itself. They have little garters too and things like that to sort of liven things up.

Maureen stressed that the safer-sex workshops she and the other facilitators conducted focused on behaviors rather than identity. This focus illustrates an unusual level of awareness of the frequent incongruence of identity and behavior. Jessie did not appear to know as much about safer sex among lesbians, and she asked technical questions. In the second group, participants first said they used dental dams for oral sex, then later said they have unsafe sex.

INTERVIEWER 2: So what about safe sex? What do lesbians do that might be unsafe, as far as when they have sex?

ALICE: Have sex with men, and then come back and have it with a woman. Don't use condoms and stuff.

INTERVIEWER 2: So what about just among women? What do two women do that might be unsafe?

RONNIE: Have unprotected sex. Really you don't know if they've been with another man.

INTERVIEWER 2: What if they've not ever been with a man?

VAL: But how do we know that, just by them telling us?

INTERVIEWER 2: But does it matter that they've ever been with a man? I mean, what if they've only been with women all their lives? Does it matter?

VAL and ?: No.

INTERVIEWER 2: So do you all use protection?

?: Yes, dental dams.

ALICE: I like—they did have the flavors. Like bubble gum or something. Strawberry's my favorite.

RONNIE: Strawberry freak, right there.

INTERVIEWER 1: So where do you get dental dams?

ALICE: When they came out to the place, out to the house, they had a AIDS thing out there. They was giving them out, condoms and those.

RONNIE: But you can get them from the hospital. Clinics will give them to you.

INTERVIEWER 1: We'll give you dental dams.

ALICE: 'Preciate that. You got any flavors?

INTERVIEWER 2: We have flavored condoms that you can cut and use.

ALICE: Cool. Strawberry?

INTERVIEWER 2: It's mint.

ALICE: That'll work.

RONNIE: We'll get you some of that strawberry preserves, okay?

ALICE: Cool Whip, get Cool Whip, too, it'll be all right.

INTERVIEWER 2: They have flavored oils though. So have any of you all had unsafe lesbian sex?

ALICE and RONNIE: Yes.

INTERVIEWER 2: Tell me about it.

RONNIE: It was good.

FANNIE: She said brain-smashing.

INTERVIEWER 2: Did you use a condom on a toy, or . . . ?

ALICE and RONNIE: Oral sex.

INTERVIEWER 2: And you didn't use a dental dam or condom?

RONNIE: No. But I did have myself checked. Clean.

INTERVIEWER 3: Do you normally?

RONNIE: No, it was just that time.

INTERVIEWER 2: What about the rest of you?

ALICE: Same.

INTERVIEWER 2: Just oral sex?

ALICE: Yeah.

INTERVIEWER 1: What about like sharing dildos without using a condom?

ALICE: No, what I have is mine. You got to get your own. I don't like to share mine like that.

INTERVIEWER 2: Where did y'all find out how to have safe lesbian sex?

VAL: I found out in jail.

ALICE: You know, we used to go to the gay parades and stuff in Atlanta, and I know some friends of mine that been gays, like I know an old woman, she's like sixty something years old. She taught me a lot. "You know, baby, you got to get them condoms, and don't let nobody use your dildo, I'm telling you. It'll fuck you up." She took me in the house. Man, she had one from like, that longest one I seen was like, I'm saying like, "Damn, granny, you use that?"

INTERVIEWER 1: So what about in jail?

VAL: That was just . . . they had a class come in.

ALICE and RONNIE: Yeah.

RONNIE: I've been to those things.

INTERVIEWER 2: In jail?

RONNIE: Yeah.

INTERVIEWER 1: What do they say? I mean, because you're not supposed to be having sex in jail, but they talk . . .

ALICE: They know you having it. You got a cellmate, ain't nobody but you and her in there. You know when guard makes rounds, by the time guard makes rounds, she got you, and he'd be asleep, it'd be on. You be too tired to do anything but brush your teeth, lay down.

This group of women knew where to get dental dams and condoms, and they knew how to use them. They also seemed aware of risk. They were aware and educated through public health avenues, such as jail and clinics, and through other people they knew, and they still did not consistently use protection. The third group briefly described their concerns regarding HIV and STIs.

INTERVIEWER 1: We are running out of tape, but there is one question that I wanted to talk about and that is how do you all feel about safe sex?

INTERVIEWER 2: Since that's what this study's about, maybe—maybe we should slip something in at the end.

INTERVIEWER 1: Are you concerned about STDs? If you are, do you practice safe sex? Or you are concerned, but not concerned enough to practice safe sex?

POLLY: I'm not concerned, but primarily because I've been in a relationship for several years. Thanks to that study, though, where I couldn't answer some of those questions, I made a promise to myself that if I in fact find myself on the loose, so to speak, I will make sure that I pay attention. Because I pay attention to everything else, I do self-exams, I get a pap done and all that stuff, but I definitely would practice safe sex if I find myself out of this particular relationship.

INTERVIEWER 1: Good for you.

EMMA: I guess ditto to what she said, because, yeah, I walked in and not being able to answer the questions very well or at all.

POLLY: Wasn't it embarrassing? I thought I knew a lot.

EMMA: Well, back when I was worried about it, we had syphilis and gonorrhea, and that was it. So yeah, I would be a little bit more aware, and inquisitive about their history, and not be offended if they ask me.

IMANI: I'm pretty damn aware. I would say I'm safe one hundred percent of the time. I do not have—I do not engage in unsafe sexual activity. Because of the nature of my relationships. I'm really into piercing, so there's always—when you get into playing with people's blood, there's always a risk of HIV.

INTERVIEWER 2: Are you into—like, you do the piercing or you get pierced?

IMANI: Both. So I would say, and I'm always like super safe when I do that, engage in that kind of activity. Just because I have, I taught safe-sex classes for AIDS projects for two years, so I'm pretty, you know, you can't ever—it's hard to be one hundred percent sure all the time, so I'm always safe. Maybe because safer sex is not safe sex, the only safe sex is abstinence, so when you're talking about safer sex, latex barrier is ninety-nine percent, but it's not one hundred percent of the time. I mean there's always a chance, so I'm really careful about that. I get tested every three months for just about everything, especially HIV/AIDS. I had—working in a HIV/AIDS ministry in my church, and my father having been a hospice nurse for years upon years, I have known so many people who have and have had HIV who have died—countless, countless number of people—that it's just, I don't ever play unsafe. I don't go there with that. It's like a hard limit with me, you know, even with my girl-friend, whatever. There is no such thing as unsafe sex in my world. It's one thing if you're monogamous, if you decide to be like fluid bonded with somebody after like two years or whatever, that's like a commitment that you want to make, and you've both been safe and tested, and tested again. My girlfriend's father died of AIDS, and I've just seen so many people die it's not worth it to not be safe.

INTERVIEWER 2: So has anybody ever objected to you wanting to use . . . ?

IMANI: Yes.

INTERVIEWER 1: What happened?

IMANI: I said, "Okay, bye. Then you're not sleeping with me." That's the end of the story, I don't do that.

INTERVIEWER 1: Did she have reasons for objecting to that?

IMANI: Most people are like, "You can't get HIV from lesbian sex." And that's BS.

Polly, like others, felt safe in the context of her current relation-ship. She felt protected by intimacy as well as by her own careful and cautious nature. Imani, like Maureen in the first group, had conducted safer-sex classes and was very certain of her own limits on risk, to the point of refusing to have what she considered to be unsafe sex. Imani showed clarity and commitment to safer sex. She says she will not consider unsafe sex: "There's no such thing as unsafe sex in my world." This certitude is derived from her expert knowledge as a safer-sex educator and from her personal experiences of watching people she cared for dying after contracting HIV. Imani's strong and unwavering line of protective action serves as a contrast to the gener-ally held belief that lesbians are at lower risk. Imani is highly aware and protective. She broke through many of the barriers to self-protec-tion described in this study. Through education and life experiences, her frame of susceptibility encompassed awareness and protection. In talking about risk, these women located risk in elements of their own lives. Those with unusual circumstances, such as the HIV activists, the virologist, and those who had spent time in jail, could not view risk solely through the frame of being a lesbian, which can connote invulnerability. These women's additional knowledge served as a prod toward protective actions. Lesbian women locate issues of risk and protection in the wider context of their lived experience of community, politics, power, and love.

Chapter 6

Discussion

Lesbian women construct and label their identities and actions in complex ways. I have examined their constructions of identity and actions, their interpretive frames of susceptibility, and their perceptions of risk and protection. I have also analyzed the barriers they face as they consider utilizing protective actions. Respondents based their choice of sexual-identity label on a number of factors that included, but were not limited to, sexual actions. Other factors were politics, group affiliation, desire, emotions, and the meaning of the label. Women who identify as lesbian do not always have sex exclusively with women. There are several contexts for this identity-divergent behavior. One is the process of coming out. Often, women have sex with men on their journey toward identifying as lesbian. As part of a larger cultural socialization, women are guided toward heterosexuality. Lesbians also may have sex with men for pleasure. Sometimes, they fall in love with men. The definition of a lesbian as a woman who has sex only with women can clash with the reality that lesbians do have sex with men. This identity divergence can serve as a barrier to protection, both for the individual for whom the divergence occurs and for those who make assumptions about a partner's behavior based on her label.

Other barriers to protection included institutional influences, such as a lack of medical and health research on lesbian women, unknowledgeable health care practitioners, and dissemination of misleading health information. Interpersonal barriers included a lack of communication, dishonesty, and lack of trust. Circumstantial barriers included engaging in sex while using alcohol or drugs, with the accompanying loosening of inhibitions, and sex exchange.

This study addresses several of the research priorities identified by the Institute of Medicine. It adds to the understanding of the actual health status of lesbian women. Although the sample was not representative, the descriptive data help illuminate the sexual health status of lesbian women. It examines and provides an exploratory explanation of lesbian-specific health risks and protective factors. These risk and protective factors were perceived by the women to be both sex related and non–sex related. The Institute of Medicine called for better definitions of sexual orientation and the meaning of lesbian sexual identity, and this study contributes to that knowledge. In this study, I examined how lesbian women construct their identity and how identity shapes their constructions of susceptibility and risk.

FINDINGS IN THEIR CONTEXT

Three interpretive frames of susceptibility emerged from this study. These frames combined with individual interpretation of meaning and context to inform respondents' constructions of susceptibility. These frames include invulnerable, aware and protective, and aware in the abstract. In many ways, the findings of this study support previous research findings. Stevens (1994a) found a cultural construction of immunity to HIV among WSWs, which is supported in this study by the frame of invulnerability many women adopted with regard to their construction of susceptibility. Stevens also found inconsistent use of safer-sex strategies, which was also found in the present study. Perry (1995) found that WSWs were not aware of the risks associated with unprotected sex with a woman. In this study, those women who were not aware of potential risks tended to fall into the category of invulnerable.

One barrier to protection is alcohol or drug use. Research has shown that alcohol and drugs play a role in sexual risk taking (Stevens, 1994a; Perry, 1995; Leigh and Stall, 1993; Young et al., 2000). Drug and alcohol use were found to be a barrier to utilizing protective actions in this study. Drug and alcohol use can lower one's inhibitions and contribute to unsafe behaviors such as engaging in sex with someone one does not know well or engaging in unprotected sex. In this study, drug use was common. Eighty-three percent of respondents had used marijuana, 42 percent had used cocaine, 32 percent had used crack, 33 percent had used speed, and 11 percent had used heroin. Half of the heroin users and about one-third of cocaine and speed users reported that drug use made them less selective with partners.

Having unprotected sex with men can potentially put one at risk for HIV or an STI. Diamant and colleagues (1999) found that younger WSWs experimented more with sex with men than did older WSWs. In this study, one context for lesbians having sex with men was the coming-out process, during which some respondents said they had sex with men. Cochran and Mays (1996) found that lesbian women often experiment sexually with their gay male friends. They found that 26 percent of their sample had had sex with a man in the year prior to the study, and 19 percent reported sex with an MSM in the three months prior to the study. In the present study, sex with men was common. Twenty-one percent had had vaginal sex with a man in the year prior to the interview, 17 percent had had oral sex with a man in that year, and 5 percent had had anal sex with a man in the year prior. Fifteen percent had sex in the prior year with a man who might have had sex with another man.

Myer (1997) used the health belief model to analyze lesbians' beliefs and practices regarding HIV. Among the women in her sample, most participated in some actions that could potentially put them at risk. That was true for this sample, as well. Kahala (1999) also used the HBM with lesbian women. She found that lesbians were convinced they were safe and felt they were not at risk because of intuition and denial. The women in her study were aware of the risks inherent in some lesbian sexual activities but did not feel personally susceptible. This was similar to the results from this study. Intuition was one of the reasons why some women in this study felt themselves to be invulnerable. Others, like the women in Kahala's study, were aware of risks but did not feel susceptible because they denied the personal relevance of those risks.

Like Stevens (1994a), I found a cultural construction of immunity to HIV among lesbians. I discovered that this construction of immunity also extends to feelings about susceptibility to sexually transmitted infections. Like the women in Stevens's study, the women in my sample inconsistently practiced safer sex. Although Stevens found a lack of awareness as to possible HIV risk among her sample, my sample showed a high level of risk awareness. For many, though, this risk was not viewed as personally relevant.

In this study, I examined how lesbian women form frames of susceptibility with regard to HIV and STI risk. These frames are influenced by sexual identity, sexual behaviors, perceptions of risk and protection, and barriers to protection. These are not one-way relationships. Figure 6.1 shows the relationships between these concepts.

This model helps our understanding of risk, protective activities, and constructions of susceptibility in a marginalized population. To begin, sexual identity and sexual actions affect one another. The notion that sexual identity is static and always matches sexual actions is false and potentially dangerous. Sexual identity is fluid. It changes over time and varies by circumstance. The same is true for sexual actions. Sexual lines of action (e.g., sex with men) do not flow directly from sexual identities. The belief that identity labels always predict actions is false, and simplistic assumptions about a potential partner based on self-labeling alone can be a barrier to utilizing protection.

Other barriers include circumstantial barriers, such as a lack of control due to drug or alcohol use or to sex exchange. This is true not only for lesbian women but also for those in the larger society. Interpersonal issues, such as communication, also serve as barriers to protection. Communicating about sex can be uncomfortable for many people. For lesbians, asking about STIs and HIV may be particularly

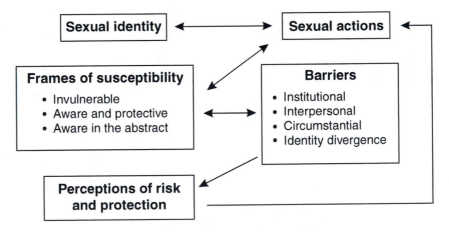

FIGURE 6.1. Frames and Barriers

problematic because of the belief that lesbians are not at risk for these. If an individual asks a potential partner about past history and STIs, she risks being stigmatized and misunderstood. Some women reported that when they tried to bring up the topic of using safer sex, their partner assumed that they had an STI. In addition, women who did have an STI sometimes hid their status from partners because of fear of potential stigma.

Institutional barriers to utilizing protection were in some ways unique to this population. Not a lot of information is available about safer sex for lesbians. What information is available may not actually get into the hands of those for whom it is intended. Traditional sex education does not cover topics of lesbian sex or lesbian protection. Health care practitioners are often themselves misinformed or uninformed as to the actual sex practices of lesbian women and whether these sex practices place lesbians at risk.

These barriers to protection have an effect on lesbian women's frames of susceptibility. If, in a particular woman's case, some barriers are missing, she may fall into the aware and protective category of susceptibility. This can be a result of obtaining clear and accurate information regarding risk and protective actions. Those women who come out to their health care practitioners have a better chance of getting good information and of putting it to use in their personal lives. Sometimes, though, health care providers do not have appropriate information. Being aware and protective can also be a result of open communication with partners and a willingness to try safer-sex techniques.

In sum, if barriers to protection are reduced, lesbians may change their view of personal susceptibility and consequently change their sexual actions. A lesbian woman's frame of susceptibility is subject to change based on a number of factors, including education, awareness, sexual identity, sexual behaviors, and perceptions of risk and protection. This shifting in stance can be permanent or situational. For example, some women did not feel a need to utilize protective actions when they had sex with a woman who identified as lesbian, but they did feel a need to utilize protective actions when their potential partner identified as bisexual. This is because of the idea that bisexual women are somehow a conduit for disease transmission from men to lesbians. Some women refuse to have sex with bisexual women.

Some bisexual women do not disclose their bisexuality, thereby depriving their partners of the choice to change their stance on risk and protection based on who they think they are having sex with.

THEORETICAL IMPLICATIONS

In this study, I used symbolic interaction and critical social constructionism to analyze data. Constructionist theory seeks to understand how people view their worlds. This study does that in that an attempt was made to view phenomena from the respondents' perspectives. I examined how lesbians construct perceptions of susceptibility, risk, and protection according to the women's stories. Identity, knowledge, and beliefs are informed by cultural affiliations and contribute to the formation of an individual's perceptions of reality. How one labels oneself and to what degree that label is internalized will affect how one constructs reality. Different individuals will interpret the same situation in different ways based on their construction of a situation, which is affected by a variety of factors. The themes that emerged from this study were generated from the respondent interviews and focus groups, and I attempted to analyze these themes with the women's perspectives in mind.

The literature on sexual identity formation shows that many factors may influence an individual's internalization and disclosure of identity (Eliason, 1996). These may include self-perceptions regarding identity and behavior, as well as the perceptions of others. This idea held true in the present study. Other studies found that sexual identity is fluid among lesbians. The women in this study corroborated that. Their constructions of identity changed over time, and this change did not take place in only one direction. For some women, their identities moved from heterosexual to bisexual to lesbian and stayed there. For others, identity shifted according to circumstance. For example, some women called themselves lesbians when they were involved with women and bisexuals when they were involved with men, and this shifted back and forth depending on their situation.

Sexual-identity formation is often viewed only within the context of self-labeling (Cox and Gallois, 1996), without attention to factors such as social interaction and interpersonal relationships. My model does take into account interpersonal factors and interaction factors. Interactions include those with health care practitioners, other individuals, the lesbian community, and the larger social world.

Individuals tend to take many aspects of their realities for granted (Berger and Luckman, 1967). For example, there is a generally held belief that lesbians are not susceptible to HIV or STIs. This group-held knowledge is shared. When a woman identifies as a lesbian and perceives herself as being part of that group, she often ends up subscribing to a body of knowledge that is at once vast, supportive, and potentially dangerous. This knowledge is often taken for granted as objective fact without further investigation. Knowledge guides people's conduct in everyday life. So if a lesbian feels she is not susceptible to HIV or STIs, she will act in accordance with that belief and will not take protective actions, because, according to the cultural beliefs, she does not need to.

Social stocks of knowledge (Schutz, 1962; Berger and Luckman, 1967) allow people to make assumptions about others and to carve out meaningful lines of actions based on these assumptions. People act in relation to a set of meanings (Blumer, 1969), and these meanings arise from social interactions and experiences. For the women in this study, this was true. Their sexual practices and interpersonal decisions are shaped by sets of meanings. These meanings included what constituted lesbian identity and behavior, what actions might be perceived as risky, and what it means to be bisexual. Lesbian identity often did mean that a woman has sex only with women. For some women, however, the label of lesbian did not preclude having sex with men. Constructions of susceptibility were influenced by interactions and experiences, but they were also influenced by membership in the group of "lesbians."

Snow (2001) emphasizes the importance of symbolization and argues that meanings are not necessarily individually constructed. Rather, meanings can come to an individual through an existing cultural condition. In this sense, interpretive frameworks (Goffman, 1974) also exist at the group level, where they often become taken for granted. When a woman decides she is a lesbian, she faces an array of existing interpretive frameworks that are available for her use. Women in this sample described several interpretive frames with regard to susceptibility. The frame of invulnerability, in particular, is a strongly held community belief. It is, in fact, often taken as a point of pride and a justification for not utilizing protective actions. Those who view their personal susceptibility through the lens of this interpretive frame are not likely to see themselves as being at risk and are not likely to utilize protective actions.

Preexisting frames are not only keyed (Goffman, 1974), brought into the discussion, or used as taken-for-granted meanings, and are not only fabricated by individuals during interaction. They are also assembled and reassembled in communities as new information and constructs spread and become part of the new wisdom and new stock of knowledge. Hence, the idea that lesbians are at greater risk than previously thought erodes the symbolic shell of "cosmic protection." We can see this in the shifting of interpretive frames that some women discussed in this study. For those who do have HIV or an STI, stigma management (Goffman, 1963) becomes important. One implication is that although nondisclosure can prevent the spoiling of identity among the discreditable in their partnerships and sexual relationships, it can also inhibit the more cautious lines of action (Blumer, 1969) associated with risk reduction.

This study also has implications for our understanding and application of the HBM. This model relates how an individual constructs health risks and susceptibility. The HBM views actions from an individual perspective. In this study, perceived susceptibility is the degree to which an individual considers herself to be at risk for HIV or STIs. Previous research has shown the perceived susceptibility of lesbians to HIV and STIs to be generally low, which has been backed up by this study. According to the HBM, if individuals have accurate knowledge regarding risks, then they will view themselves as being susceptible (if they are susceptible) and will take steps to utilize protective measures and minimize risk. Likelihood of behavior change is dependent on perceived susceptibility, perceived threat of the disease, and barriers to protection. Cues to action also are important, and these include education, personal experience, and beliefs (Kiser, 1990).

In the case of lesbians and HIV and STIs, things are not that simple. Constructions of susceptibility are affected not only by knowledge but also by ideas and cultural themes that exist outside of the individual and that have a life of their own. Of course, that knowledge is not always available, nor is it always accurate. When an individual's identity shifts, her interpretive framework may shift as well. This can be long term and enduring or short term and situational. The HBM may not be useful as it stands in evaluating risks for this group. It should include a more explicit recognition of an individual's group placement, along with an understanding of the assumptions and interpretive frameworks associated with that group.

APPLIED IMPLICATIONS

This study has several applied implications. These include the following:

Health Implications

- Lesbian health care–seeking behavior
- Lesbian sexual risk and protection

Medical Implications

- Education for practitioners
- Recommendations for practitioners with lesbian and bisexual patients

Educational Implications

- Safer-sex materials
- Sex education
- Community education

Media

- Dissemination of accurate materials
- Lesbian media depiction of risk and protection

Policy Implications

- Institute of Medicine recommendations
- Inclusion of variety of experiences

- Inclusion of variety of standpoints in health policy formation
- Research funding

Recommendations for Further Research

- Include wide variety in sampling to include variety of experiences and viewpoints
- Further investigation of the meanings of labels and label choice
- Further investigation of the relationship between identity and behavior
- Further investigation of interpretive frames and community-held beliefs
- Development and use of standard measures for identity and behavior

This study provides information on lesbian women's sexual identity and actions that can be useful in helping these women understand some of the beliefs and practices of others in their community. It is important to help women make more-informed choices as to their own sexual practices. The first area is in their health care–seeking behavior. It is clear that everyone, regardless of sexual identity, should be as candid and comprehensive as possible in disclosing health-related information to their health care providers. This means that lesbians should disclose their sexuality to their doctors in situations in which it is relevant. This includes general exams and gynecological visits. Such disclosure can help their doctors ask the right questions and give appropriate recommendations. It will also help educate individual practitioners about lesbian lives and diversity. If a woman is not comfortable discussing her sexual identity with her practitioner, she should consider finding someone with whom she is comfortable. If a woman experiences homophobia or discrimination as a result of disclosing her sexual identity, then she should discuss this with the practitioner and also consider making a report to appropriate authorities.

Lesbian women should be getting regular pap smears. Research shows that even some lesbians who have never had sex with a man have HPV, which is thought to lead to cervical cancer. Pap exams also allow doctors to visually screen for other sexually transmitted infections or health problems which a woman might not detect on her own. Lesbian women should also consider being screened for HIV or STIs. Perhaps most important, these women should be aware of their actions and make informed choices about the risks and protective measures they choose to take. Many women already ask potential partners about their sexual history. This should be standard practice. When finding themselves in a situation defined as potentially risky, lesbian women should utilize protective behaviors. Also, lesbian women should consider HIV and STI screening for both partners at the start of a new relationship. Because many STIs lack recognizable symptoms, this screening could identify unknown problems and allow the couple to then take appropriate actions to prevent transmission.

In addition to lesbian health implications, medical implications also arose from this study. The first, and most pressing, is education for practitioners. More medical-based research should be conducted on lesbian sexual health. More studies that show or deny transmission of specific STIs should be done so that relevant recommendations can be made and appropriate treatment of patients can be planned. General practitioners, gynecologists, and others who examine women's sexual health should have special supplementary education regarding the identity and sexual practices of lesbians. They should be aware that lesbians sometimes have sex with men. They should be aware that lesbians sometimes get pregnant and give birth. They should be aware of the potential for STI or HIV transmission between lesbians, and they should be able to provide their patients with appropriate educational and safer-sex materials. They should also be aware of homophobia and the issues that accompany it, and they and their staff should be aware of their own actions in this regard.

Practitioners with lesbian and bisexual patients should develop or adopt appropriate screening forms, such as those used at many women's health centers, that ask questions about identity and actions in a nonthreatening manner. The forms should not reflect any assumptions about women's actions or biases about identity or actions. Practitioners should also make an effort to keep up with the latest research on lesbian sexual health. As this is an emerging field, research assumptions and findings change often.

Besides individual autonomous actions from lesbian women and from medical practitioners, more general educational measures are in order. Safer-sex materials that are generally available to the public almost exclusively discuss heterosexual sex. These materials should be expanded to include same-sex activities and risks (for both women and men). It would be a simple matter to add a few sentences here and there. In addition to these general safer-sex materials, more material should be available that focuses specifically on woman-to-woman sex. These materials should include mention of identity divergence and also should include some of the non-sex-related risks brought up by women in this study, such as sharing razors or toothbrushes. Sex-education materials should include sections on gay and lesbian sex. Adolescents and young adults who are becoming sexually active need to have access to accurate and current information that addresses their needs. University health centers should provide safer-sex materials and lectures on lesbian health. In addition to health centers, women's groups, both on campus and off, should include seminars on lesbian-specific health issues as well as including lesbian issues in more general women's talks.

Portrayals of lesbian women have become almost commonplace on television and in the movies. Although these characters are a great leap forward in educating the public about lesbians, there is room for more depth with regard to their lives and health issues. Women's programs that focus on sexual health should include lesbian health as part of those discussions. Magazines, both lesbian and mainstream, should pay more attention to health issues of lesbian and bisexual women. The news media can do a better job of reporting research findings on lesbian health. Currently, this occurs only in lesbian- or gay-specific news media.

Policy recommendations follow those of the Institute of Medicine. Policymakers should include a variety of experiences and lifestyles in their discussions of women's health policy. In both social and medical research, investigators should include a wider variety of study participants and not rely on the traditionally easier-to-reach subgroups. Too many studies focus on white, middle-class women, and the inattention to other groups contributes to a false picture of lesbian health. When translating research findings to policy, it is important to include different types of research conducted with different populations. Policymakers should not view all lesbian women as a uniform population with uniform needs and interests. Research funding should be allocated that specifically investigates lesbian health among all subgroups.

Research recommendations are varied. The first is to include a wide variety of experiences and types of people in sampling. I did this with targeted sampling, and in future studies I will employ the same strategies as well as more snowball sampling in the smaller subgroups. Diversity should be sought on the basis of sexual-identity labels, sexual actions, ethnicity, age, social class, and other factors such as jail or sex work. There should be further investigation into the meanings of labels and label choices. What does sexual identity mean, and how do differing meanings contribute to or detract from research and research implications? This should be investigated not just for lesbian women but for all groups. In addition, the relationship between identity and actions should be investigated for all groups. Sociologists should also investigate how the use of interpretive frames and the pervasiveness of community-held beliefs influence an individual's health-related practices. Sociologists should seek to develop standardized measures for identity and actions so that we can compare across studies and build on one another's research for a clearer understanding. We should try to use comparable sampling frames as well. Also, this study and many others lacks a fullness of interpretation by focusing only on sex and health-related issues. Other factors, such as mental health, relationships, intimate violence, sexual abuse, and so on might certainly play a role in women's risk and protective behaviors.

Appendix

Qualitative Respondents' Characteristics

Pseudonym	Age	Race	Education	STI	Sexual identity	HIV test	HIV positive
Abigail	45	white	college degree	genital herpes	lesbian	yes	no
Allison	29	white	college degree	none	lesbian	no	don't know
Amy	24	white	college degree	none	bisexual	yes	no
Andrea	25	white	college degree	none	lesbian	yes	no
Anne	35	white	grade school	trichomoniasis	lesbian	yes	no
Annette	27	white	some college	crabs	queer	yes	no
Barbara	25	white	some college	genital herpes	bisexual	yes	no
Becca	31	white	college degree	none	lesbian	yes	no
Betty	45	white	college degree	trichomoniasis	lesbian	yes	no
Bonnie	32	white	college degree	none	gay	yes	no
Brenda	33	African American	high school	none	bisexual	yes	yes
Cara	21	white	some college	none	lesbian	yes	no
Carol	36	African American	college degree	gonorrhea	other	yes	yes
Cassie	38	African American	some college	none	lesbian	no	no

Pseudonym	Age	Race	Education	STI	Sexual identity	HIV test	HIV positive
Catherine	38	white	college degree	none	lesbian	yes	no
Daphne	29	white	college degree	none	gay	yes	no
Debbie	26	white	college degree	none	lesbian	no	don't know
Ebony	23	African American	college degree	none	bisexual	yes	no
Elanor	27	white	college degree	genital herpes	lesbian	yes	no
Emily	24	white	some college	none	bisexual	yes	no
Esther	43	white	college degree	none	straight	yes	no
Frances	21	white	college degree	none	lesbian	yes	no
Gert	27	African American	college degree	none	gay	yes	no
Harriet	27	white	college degree	none	lesbian	yes	no
Heather	44	white	some college	none	lesbian	yes	no
Helen	33	African American	high school	trichomoniasis	bisexual	yes	no
Holly	24	other	college degree	none	lesbian	yes	no
Jane	24	Native American	some college	none	lesbian	yes	no
Jean	23	white	some college	none	queer	yes	no
Jennifer	28	white	college degree	genital herpes	lesbian	yes	no
Jessica	21	other	some college	none	other	no	no
Jill	26	white	some college	none	other	yes	no
Joe	26	Latina	college degree	trichomoniasis	lesbian	yes	no

Pseudonym	Age	Race	Education	STI	Sexual identity	HIV test	HIV positive
Juanita	28	African American	some college	none	lesbian	yes	no
Katie	45	white	post high school	none	gay	yes	no
Laurie	32	white	college degree	chlamydia	lesbian	yes	no
Leah	25	white	some college	none	lesbian	yes	no
Lori	22	white	some college	genital herpes	bisexual	yes	no
Lorna	33	white	high school	trichomoniasis	lesbian	yes	yes
Mai	33	Asian American	college degree	none	bisexual	yes	no
Maria	22	Latina	some college	none	lesbian	no	don't know
Mary	49	African American	college degree	none	bisexual	yes	no
Meg	28	white	some college	none	lesbian	yes	no
Michelle	24	white	college degree	none	gay	yes	no
Mindy	26	Asian American	some college	none	queer	yes	no
Monique	35	African American	high school	none	lesbian	yes	no
Nicole	38	white	college degree	none	lesbian	yes	no
Pamela	22	white	college degree	genital herpes	other	yes	no
Patty	35	white	college degree	none	queer	yes	no
Polly	33	other	some college	none	lesbian	yes	no
Rachel	32	white	college degree	none	gay	yes	no

Pseudonym	Age	Race	Education	STI	Sexual identity	HIV test	HIV positive
Robin	21	white	college degree	none	lesbian	yes	no
Sally	37	African American	college degree	none	lesbian	yes	no
Sandra	39	white	some college	none	lesbian	yes	no
Shanida	41	African American	college degree	none	lesbian	yes	no
Shawn	29	African American	some college	none	lesbian	yes	no
Stacey	23	white	college degree	genital warts/ HPV	lesbian	yes	no
Stella	28	African American	college degree	none	lesbian	yes	no
Stephanie	29	African American	some college	none	gay	yes	no
Sue	28	white	college degree	none	queer	no	don't know
Tammy	26	white	some college	none	gay	yes	no
Tanika	28	African American	high school	none	lesbian	yes	don't know
Tavis	37	African American	some college	none	lesbian	yes	no
Tawna	29	African American	college degree	none	bisexual	yes	no
Teresa	39	white	college degree	none	lesbian	yes	no
Valerie	30	white	college degree	none	lesbian	yes	no
Veronica	29	white	some college	none	lesbian	yes	no
Zelda	46	white	college degree	none	lesbian	yes	no

References

Berger, B. J., J. M. Zenilman, M. C. Cummings, J. Feldman, and W. M. McCormack (1995). "Bacterial Vaginosis in Lesbians: A Sexually Transmitted Disease." *Clinical Infectious Diseases* 21(6):1402-1405.

Berger, P. and T. Luckman (1967). *The Social Construction of Reality: A Treatise in the Sociology of Knowledge.* New York: Anchor.

Bevier, P. J., M. A. Chiasson, R. T. Hefferman, and K. G. Castro (1995). "Women at a Sexually Transmitted Disease Clinic Who Reported Same-Sex Contact: Their HIV Seroprevalence and Risk Behaviors." *American Journal of Public Health* 85(10):1366-1371.

Blumer, H. (1969). *Symbolic Interaction.* Englewood Cliffs, NJ: Prentice-Hall.

Brogan, D., E. Frank, L. Elon, and K. A. O'Hanlan (2001). "Methodologic Concerns in Defining Lesbian for Health Research." *Epidemiology* 12(1):109-113.

Cass, V. C. (1996). "Sexual Orientation Identity Formation: A Western Phenomenon." In R. P. Cabaj and T. S. Stein (Eds.), *Textbook of Homosexuality and Mental Health* (pp. 227-251). Washington, DC: American Psychiatric Press.

Caster, W. (1993). *The Lesbian Sex Book.* Los Angeles: Alyson Books.

Centers for Disease Control and Prevention (1995). "What Are Women Who Have Sex with Women's HIV Prevention Needs?" National Center for HIV, STD and TB Prevention. Division of HIV/AIDS Prevention. *Report on Lesbian HIV Issues Meeting.* Available online: <http://www.caps.ucsf.edu/capsweb/wsw.html>.

Centers for Disease Control and Prevention (1997). "HIV/AIDS and Women Who Have Sex with Women in the United States." National Center for HIV, STD and TB Prevention. Division of HIV/AIDS Prevention.

Centers for Disease Control and Prevention (1999). "HIV/AIDS and Women Who Have Sex with Women." National Center for HIV, STD and TB Prevention. Division of HIV/AIDS Prevention.

Cochran, S. and V. M. Mays (1993). "Applying Social Psychological Models to Predicting HIV-Related Sexual Risk Behaviors Among African-Americans." *Journal of Black Psychology* 19(2):142-154.

Cochran, S.D. and V.M. Mays (1996). "Prevalence of HIV-Related Sexual Risk Behaviors Among 18-to-24-year-old Lesbian and Bisexual Women." *Women's Health: Research on Gender, Behavior, and Policy* 2(1&2):75-89.

Cohen, H., M. Marmor, H. Wolfe, and D. Ribble (1993). "Risk Assessment of HIV Transmission Among Lesbians." *Journal of Acquired Immune Deficiency Syndrome* 6(10):1173-1174.

Cox, S. and C. Gallois (1996). "Gay and Lesbian Identity Development: A Social Identity Perspective." *Journal of Homosexuality* 30(4):1-30.

Cranston, K. (1992). "HIV Education for Gay, Lesbian, and Bisexual Youth: Personal Risk, Personal Power and the Community of Conscience." *Journal of Homosexuality* 22(3-4):247-259.

Dean, L., H. Meyer, K. Robinson, R. L. Sell, R. Sember, V. M. B. Silenzio, D. J. Bowden, J. Bradford, E. Rothblum, J. Scout, et al. (2000). "Lesbian, Gay, Bisexual, and Transgender Health: Findings and Concerns." *Journal of the Gay and Lesbian Medical Association* 4(3):101-151.

Denenberg, R. (1997). "HIV Risks in Women Who Have Sex With Women." *Treatment Issues* 11(7/8):25.

Deren, S., A. Estrada, M. Stark, and M. Goldstein (1999). "Sexual Orientation and HIV Risk Behaviors in a National Sample of Injection Drug Users and Crack Smokers." *Drugs and Society* 9:97-108.

Diamant, A. L., J. Lever, and M. A. Schuster (2000). "Lesbians' Sexual Activities and Efforts to Reduce Risks for Sexually Transmitted Diseases." *Journal of the Gay and Lesbian Medical Association* 4(2):41-48.

Diamant, A. L., M. A. Schuster, K. McGuigan, and J. Lever (1999). "Lesbians' Sexual History with Men: Implications for Taking a Sexual History." *Archives of Internal Medicine* 159(22):2730-2736.

Diamant, A. L., C. Wold, K. Spritzer, and L. Gelberg (2000). "Health Behaviors, Health Status, and Access to and Use of Health Care." *Archives of Family Medicine* 9:1043-1051.

Edwards, A. and R. N. Thin (1990). "Sexually Transmitted Diseases in Lesbians." *International Journal of STD and AIDS* 1:178-181.

Einhorn, L. and M. Polgar (1994). "HIV Risk Behavior Among Lesbians and Bisexual Women." *AIDS Education and Prevention* 6(6):514-523.

Eliason, M. J. (1996). *Institutional Barriers to Health Care for Lesbian, Gay, and Bisexual Persons.* New York: NLN Press.

Faderman, L. (1984). "The 'New Gay' Lesbians." *Journal of Homosexuality* 10(3/4):85-95.

Fethers, K., C. Marks, A. Mindel, and C. S. Estcourt (2000). "Sexually Transmitted Infections and Risk Behaviours in Women Who Have Sex with Women." *Sexually Transmitted Infections* 76:345-349.

Fishbein, M. and M. Guinan (1996). "Behavioral Science and Public Health: A Necessary Partnership for HIV Prevention." *Public Health Reports* 111:5-10.

Georgia Department of Human Resources (2001). "Quarterly HIV/AIDS Surveillance Reports." Available online: <http://georgiaaidsinfoline.com/gastat101.htm>.

Gielen, A. C., R. R. Faden, P. O'Campo, N. Kass, and J. Anderson (1994). "Women's Protective Sexual Behaviors: A Test of the Health Belief Model." *AIDS Education and Prevention* 6(1):1-11.

Glanz, K., F. M. Lewis, and B. K. Rimer (1997). *Health Behavior and Health Education: Theory, Research, and Practice.* San Francisco: Jossey-Bass.

Glaser, B. and A. Strauss (1967). *The Discovery of Grounded Theory: Strategies for Qualitative Research.* New York: Aldine de Gruyter.

Goffman, E. (1963). *Stigma: Notes on the Management of Spoiled Identities.* Englewood Cliffs, NJ: Prentice-Hall.

Goffman, E. (1974). *Frame Analysis: An Essay on the Organization of Experience.* New York: Harper Colophon.

Grossman, A. H. (1994). "Homophobia: A Cofactor of HIV Disease in Gay and Lesbian Youth." *Journal of the Association of Nurses in AIDS Care* 5(1):39-43.

Hastie, B. (2000). "Of Dykes and Data." *Poz.* February, p. 53.

Heffernan, K. (1998). "The Nature and Predictors of Substance Use Among Lesbians." *Addictive Behaviors* 23(4):517-528.

Henry, S. (2001). "Constructionist Theory." In C. D. Bryant (Ed.), *Encyclopedia of Criminology and Deviant Behavior* (pp. 52-55). Philadelphia: Brunner-Routledge.

Hunter, S., C. Shannon, J. Knox, and J. I. Martin (1998). *Lesbian, Gay and Bisexual Youths and Adults: Knowledge for Human Services Practice.* Thousand Oaks, CA: Sage Publications.

Kahala, O. (1999). "Perception of HIV Infection Risk Among Lesbians and Gay Men." Presented at the 1999 American Sociological Association Meeting.

Kaplan, C. D., D. Korf, and C. Sterk (1987). "Temporal and Social Contexts of Heroin-Using Populations: An Illustration of the Snowball Sampling Technique." *Journal of Nervous and Mental Disease* 175(9):566-574.

Kennedy, M. B., M. I. Scarlett, A. C. Duerr, and S. Y. Chu (1995). "Assessing HIV Risk Among Women Who Have Sex with Women: Scientific and Communication Issues." *Journal of the American Medical Women's Association* 50(3/4):103-107.

Kirk, J. and M. Miller (1985). *Reliability and Validity in Qualitative Research.* Newbury Park, CA: Sage Publications.

Kiser, M. (1990). "Predicting Preventive Health Behavior: The Health Belief Model." Master's thesis, Department of Sociology, Georgia State University, Atlanta.

Kral, A. H., J. Lorvick, R. N. Bluthenthal, and J. K. Watters (1997). "HIV Risk Profile of Drug-Using Women Who Have Sex with Women in 19 United States Cities." *Journal of Acquired Immune Deficiency Syndromes and Human Retrovirology* 16:211-217.

Krauss, B. J., L. Goldsamt, E. Bula, and R. Sember (1997). "The White Researcher in the Multicultural Community: Lessons in HIV Prevention Education Learned in the Field." *Journal of Health Education* 28(6):67-71.

Leifer, C. and E. W. Young (1997). "Homeless Lesbians: Psychology of the Hidden, the Disenfranchised, and the Forgotten." *Journal of Psychosocial Nursing* 35(10):28-33.

Leigh, B. C. and R. Stall (1993). "Substance Use and Risky Sexual Behavior for Exposure to HIV." *American Psychologist* 48(10):1035-1045.

Lemp, G. F., M. Jones, T. A. Kellog, G. N. Nieri, L. Anderson, D. Withum, and M. Katz (1995). "HIV Seroprevalence and Risk Behaviors among Lesbians and

Bisexual Women in San Francisco and Berkeley, California." *American Journal of Public Health* 85(10):1549-1552.

Maguen, S. and L. Armistead (2000). "Prevalence of Unprotected Sex and HIV-Antibody Testing Among Gay, Lesbian, and Bisexual Youth." *Journal of Sex Research* 37(2):169-174.

Magura, S., J. O'Day, and A. Rosenblum (1992). "Women Usually Take Care of Their Girlfriends: Bisexuality and HIV Risk Among Female Intravenous Drug Users." *The Journal of Drug Issues* 22(1):179-190.

Marble, M. and K. K. Key (1996). "Sexual Transmission of BV Confirmed in Lesbian Study Group." *Infectious Disease Weekly,* January 29, pp. 7-9.

Marrazzo, J. M. (2000a). "Genital Human Papillomavirus Infection in Women Who Have Sex with Women: A Concern for Patients and Providers." *AIDS Patient Care and STDs* 14(8):447-451.

Marrazzo, J. M. (2000b). "Sexually Transmitted Infections in Women Who Have Sex with Women: Who Cares?" *Sexually Transmitted Infections* 76(5):330-332.

Marrazzo, J. M., L. A. Koutsky, and H. H. Handsfield (2001). "Characteristics of Female Sexually Transmitted Disease Clinic Clients Who Report Same-Sex Behavior." *International Journal of STD and AIDS* 12(1):41-46.

McCaffrey, M., P. Varney, B. Evans, and D. Taylor-Robinson (1999). "Bacterial Vaginosis in Lesbians: Evidence for Lack of Sexual Transmission." *International Journal of STD and AIDS* 10(5):305-308.

Morrow, K. (1996). "Culture-Specific HIV/STD Prevention Programming for Lesbian and Bisexual Women." Doctoral dissertation, Department of Psychology, Western Michigan University, Kalamazoo.

Morrow, K. M. and J. E. Allsworth (2000). "Sexual Risk in Lesbians and Bisexual Women." *Journal of the Gay and Lesbian Medical Association* 4(4):159-165.

Morse, J. M. and P. A. Field (1995). *Qualitative Research Methods for Health Professionals.* Thousand Oaks, CA: Sage Publications.

Myer, L. L. (1997). "Lesbians and HIV/AIDS: The Clean and the Free?" Master's thesis, Department of Social Work, University of Nevada, Reno.

Nation's Health (1995). "AMA Adopts Policy on Gay, Lesbian Health." *Nation's Health* 25(1):20.

Norman, A. D., M. J. Perry, L. Y. Stevenson, J. A. Kelly, and R. A. Roffman (1996). "Lesbian and Bisexual Women in Small Cities—At Risk for HIV?" *Public Health Reports* 111:347-352.

Pederson, W. B. (1994). "HIV Risk in Gay and Lesbian Adolescents." *Journal of Gay and Lesbian Social Services* 1(3-4):131-147.

Perry, S. M. (1994). "Prediction of Risky Sexual Behaviors Among Lesbians: A Theoretical Comparison." Doctoral dissertation, Department of Psychology, University of Houston, Texas.

Perry, S. M. (1995). "Lesbian Alcohol and Marijuana Use: Correlates of HIV Risk Behaviors and Abusive Relationships." *Journal of Psychoactive Drugs* 27(4):13-19.

Potter, J. (1999). "Should Sexual Partners of Women with Bacterial Vaginosis Receive Treatment?" *British Journal of General Practice* 49:913-918.

Quah, S. R. (1998). "Ethnicity, HIV/AIDS Prevention and Public Health Education." *International Journal of Sociology and Social Policy* 18(7/8):1-23.

Raiteri, R., I. Baussano, M. Giobbia, R. Fora, and A. Sinico (1998). "Lesbian Sex and Risk of HIV Transmission." *AIDS* 12(4):450-451.

Raiteri, R., R. Fora, L. P. Goannin, R. Russo, L. A. Lucchin, M. G. Terzi, D. Giacobbi, and A. Sinico (1994). "Seroprevalence, Risk Factors and Attitude to HIV-1 in a Representative Sample of Lesbians in Turin." *Genitourinary Medicine* 70:200-205.

Raiteri, R., R. Fora, and A. Sinico (1994). "HIV Risk Found 'Non-Existent' Among Lesbians" [News]. *Nursing Times* 90(31):10-11.

Rankow, E. J. (1995). "Lesbian Health Issues for the Primary Care Provider." *The Journal of Family Practice* 40(5):486-492.

Reynolds, G. (1994). "HIV and Lesbian Sex." *The Lancet* 344:544-545.

Richters, J., S. Lubowitz, S. Bergin, and G. Prestage (1998). "HIV Risks Among Women in Contact With Sydney's Gay and Lesbian Community." *Venereology* 11(3):35-38.

Robertson, P. and J. S. Schachter (1981). "Failure to Identify Venereal Disease in a Lesbian Population." *Sexually Transmitted Diseases* April-June:75-76.

Rochman, S. (1999). "Between Women." *The Advocate,* May 25, pp. 73-74.

Rothblum, E. D. (2000). "Comments on 'Lesbians'' Sexual Activities and Efforts to Reduce Risks for Sexually Transmitted Diseases." *Journal of the Gay and Lesbian Medical Association* 4(2):39-40.

Saunders, J. M. (1999). "Health Problems of Lesbian Women." *Nursing Clinics of North America* 34(2):381-391.

Savage, Dan (2001). "Savage Love" [Online advice column]. September 9. <http://www.thestranger.com/2001-09-06/savage.html>.

Schramm-Evans, Z. (1995). *Making Out: The Book of Lesbian Sex and Sexuality.* London: Pandora.

Schutz, A. (1962). *Collected Papers,* Volume 1. The Hague: Martinus Nijoff.

Shotsky, W. J. (1996). "Women Who Have Sex with Other Women: HIV Seroprevalence in New York Counseling and Testing Programs." *Women and Health* 24(2):1-15.

Smith, E. M., S. R. Johnson, and S. M. Guenther (1985). "Health Care Attitudes and Experiences During Gynecological Care Among Lesbians and Bisexuals." *American Journal of Public Health* 75(9):1085-1087.

Snow, D. A. (2001). "Extending and Broadening Blumer's Conceptualization of Symbolic Interaction." *Symbolic Interaction* 24(3):367-377.

Solarz, A. L. (Ed.) (1999). *Lesbian Health: Current Assessment and Directions for the Future.* Washington, DC: National Academy Press.

Stevens, P. E. (1993). "Lesbians and HIV: Clinical, Research and Policy Issues." *American Journal of Orthopsychiatry* 63(2):289-294.

Stevens, P. E. (1994a). "HIV Prevention Education for Lesbians and Bisexual Women: A Cultural Analysis of a Community Intervention." *Social Science and Medicine* 29:1565-1578.

Stevens, P. E. (1994b). "Lesbians' Health-Related Experiences of Care and Noncare." *Western Journal of Nursing Research* 16(6):639-659.

Strauss, A. and J. Corbin (1990). *Basics of Qualitative Research: Grounded Theory Process and Techniques.* Newbury Park, CA: Sage Publications.

Strecher, V. J. and I. M. Rosenstock (1997). "The Health Belief Model." In K. Glanz, F. M. Lewis, and B. K. Rimer (Eds.), *Health Behavior and Health Education: Theory, Research and Practice* (pp. 41-59). San Francisco: Jossey-Bass Publishers.

Taylor, B. (1999). "'Coming Out' As a Life Transition: Homosexual Identity Formation and Its Implications for Health Care Practice." *Journal of Advanced Nursing* 30(2):520-525.

Travers, R. and D. Paoletti (1999). "Responding to the Support Needs of HIV Positive Lesbian, Gay and Bisexual Youth." *Canadian Journal of Human Sexuality* 8(4):271-285.

Troiden, R. R. (1989). "The Formation of Homosexual Identities." *Journal of Homosexuality* 17(1/2):43-73.

Tronosco, A. R., A. Romani, C. M. Carranza, J. R. Macias, and R. Masini (1995). "Probable Transmission of HIV by Female Homosexual Contact" [In Spanish]. *Medicina* 55:334-336.

Walters, M. C. and W. G. Rector (1986). "Sexual Transmission of Hepatitis A in Lesbians." *Journal of the American Medical Association* 265(5):594.

Waters, M. (1994). *Modern Sociological Theory.* Thousand Oaks, CA: Sage Publications.

Watters, J. and P. Biernacki (1989). "Targeted Sampling: Options for the Study of Hidden Populations." *Social Problems* 6:416-430.

Whetsell, C. J. (1990). "The Relationship of Beliefs About AIDS to Knowledge About AIDS in Three Groups of Female Inmates (General Population, IV Drug Using, and HIV positive)." Doctoral dissertation, Department of Counseling Psychology, University of Kentucky, Lexington.

White, J. C. and W. Levinson (1995). "Lesbian Health Care: What a Primary Physician Needs to Know." *Western Journal of Medicine* 162:463-466.

Williamson, I. R. (2000). "Internalized Homophobia and Health Issues Affecting Lesbians and Gay Men." *Health Education Research* 15(1):97-107.

Wilton, T. (1997). *Good for You: A Handbook on Lesbian Health and Wellbeing.* London: Cassell.

Yep, G. (1993). "Health Beliefs and HIV Prevention: Do They Predict Monogamy and Condom Use?" *Journal of Social Behavior and Personality* 8(3):507-520.

Young, R. M., S. Friedman, P. Case, M. W. Asencio, and M. Clatts (2000). "Women Injection Drug Users Who Have Sex with Women Exhibit Increased HIV Infection and Risk Behaviors." *Journal of Drug Issues* 30(3):499-534.

Young, R. M., G. Weissman, and J. Cohen (1992). "Assessing Risk in the Absence of Information: HIV Risk Among Women Injection-Drug Users Who Have Sex with Women." *AIDS and Public Policy Journal* 7:175-183.

Index